T0100152

DRUG DEVELOPMENT AND RARE PEDIATRIC DISEASES

ISSUES, STRATEGIC PLAN, AND VOUCHER PROGRAM ASSESSMENT

PHARMACOLOGY - RESEARCH, SAFETY TESTING AND REGULATION

Additional books in this series can be found on Nova's website under the Series tab.

Additional e-books in this series can be found on Nova's website under the eBooks tab.

DRUG DEVELOPMENT AND RARE PEDIATRIC DISEASES

ISSUES, STRATEGIC PLAN, AND VOUCHER PROGRAM ASSESSMENT

FREDERICK JOHNSTON
EDITOR

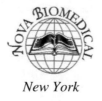

New York

NOTICE TO THE READER

Library of Congress Cataloging-in-Publication Data

ISBN: 978-1-53610-227-7

Published by Nova Science Publishers, Inc. † New York

CONTENTS

PREFACE

Over the past few decades, a number of legislative actions have been taken to encourage the development of therapies to treat people affected by rare diseases and to encourage therapies for pediatric patients. During this same time period, the Food and Drug Administration (FDA) has invested substantial effort in support of these same goals. As described in this book, recent legislative actions have prompted new initiatives. Continuing the response to the laws' specific requirements and FDA's commitment under PDUFA, this book includes input from the public and FDA and discusses the many complex issues involved in medical product development for people with rare diseases. Following a brief overview of both legislative and FDA efforts over the years to foster development of therapies for these patients, the book summarizes the three days of the public meeting and presents FDA's strategic plan for accelerating the development of the urgently needed therapies for pediatric rare diseases.

In: Drug Development   ISBN: 978-1-53610-227-7
Editor: Frederick Johnston   © 2016 Nova Science Publishers, Inc.

Chapter 1

REPORT: COMPLEX ISSUES IN DEVELOPING DRUGS AND BIOLOGICAL PRODUCTS FOR RARE DISEASES AND ACCELERATING THE DEVELOPMENT OF THERAPIES FOR PEDIATRIC RARE DISEASES INCLUDING STRATEGIC PLAN: ACCELERATING THE DEVELOPMENT OF THERAPIES FOR PEDIATRIC RARE DISEASES[*]

Food and Drug Adminstration

LIST OF ABBREVIATIONS

ABBREVIATION	DEFINITION
ADEPT	Advancing the Development of Pediatric Therapies
ADN	Annual Distribution Number
BLA	Biologic License Application
BPCA	Best Pharmaceuticals for Children Act
CBER	Center for Biologics Evaluation and Research
CDER	Center for Drug Evaluation and Research

---

[*] This is an edited, reformatted and augmented version of a report issued by the FDA, July 2014.

(Continued)

ABBREVIATION	DEFINITION
CDRH	Center for Devices and Radiological Health
CFSAN	Center for Food Safety and Applied Nutrition
CMS	Centers for Medicare and Medicaid Services
COA	Clinical Outcome Assessment
CPIM	Critical Path Innovation Meeting
DDT	Drug Development Took
DGIEP	Division of Gastroenterology and Inborn Errors Products
EAP	Expedited Access PMA
EMA	European Medicines Agency
ETASU	Elements to Assure Safe Use
FDA	Food and Drug Administration
FDAAA	Food and Drug Administration Amendments Act
FDASIA	Food and Drug Administration Safety and Innovation Act
FD&C Act	Federal Food, Drug, and Cosmetic Act
HDE	Humanitarian Device Exemption
HIV	Human Immunodeficiency Virus
HUD	Humanitarian Use Device
IDE	Investigational Device Exemption
IMM	Irreversible Morbidity or Mortality
IND	Investigational New Drug Application
IOM	Institute of Medicine
IPA	Intergovernmental Personnel Act
IRDiRC	International Rare Diseases Research Consortium
MDIC	Medical Device Innovation Consortium
NAM	Nonclinical Assessment Models
NCATS	National Center for Advancing Translational Sciences
NCTR	National Center for Toxicological Research
NDA	New Drug Application
NICHD	Eunice Kennedy Shriver National Institute of Child Health and Human Development
NIH	National Institutes of Health
NME	New Molecular Entity
NORD	National Organization for Rare Disorders
OCOMM	Office of Communications
OCTGT	Office of Cellular, Tissue and Gene Therapies

ABBREVIATION	DEFINITION
ODA	Orphan Drug Act
OHCA	Office of Health and Constituent Affairs
OHOP	Office of Hematology and Oncology Products
OOPD	Office of Orphan Products Development
OPD	Orphan Products Development
OPP	Office of Policy and Planning
OPT	Office of Pediatric Therapeutics
OND	Office of New Drugs
ORISE	Oak Ridge Institute for Science and Education
OSEL	Office of Science and Engineering Laboratories
OTS	Office of Translational Sciences
PBPK	Physiologically-Based Pharmacokinetic
PCORI	Patient Centered Outcome Research Institute
PDC	Pediatric Device Consortia
PDUFA	Prescription Drug User Fee Act
PeRC	Pediatric Review Committee
POD	Pharmacokinetic/Pharmacodynamics
PMA	Premarket Approval
PMDSIA	Pediatric Medical Device Safety and improvement Act
PMHS	Pediatric and Maternal Health Staff
PRD	Pediatric Rare Diseases
PREA	Pediatric Research Equity Act
PRO	Patient Reported Outcome
PRV	Priority Review Voucher
PSP	Pediatric Study Plan
RDP	Rare Disease Program
REMS	Risk Evaluation and Mitigation Strategy
SEALD	Study Endpoints and Labeling Development
TP LC	Total Product Life Cycle

EXECUTIVE SUMMARY

Purpose and Background

Over the past few decades, a number of legislative actions have been taken to encourage the development of therapies to treat people affected by rare diseases and to encourage therapies for pediatric patients. During this same time period, the Food and Drug Administration (FDA) has invested substantial effort in support of these same goals. As described in this report, recent legislative actions have prompted new initiatives.

In 2012, the U.S. Congress passed the Food and Drug Administration Safety and Innovation Act (FDASIA)[1], which requires FDA to hold a public meeting to discuss ways to encourage and accelerate the development of new therapies for pediatric rare diseases, and to issue a report that includes a strategic plan for encouraging and accelerating such therapies.[2]

FDASIA also includes the fifth authorization of the Prescription Drug User Fee Act (PDUFA), under which FDA agreed to conduct a public meeting to discuss complex issues in clinical trials for studying drugs for rare diseases and to make a summary of that meeting available publicly through the FDA website.[3]

In view of shared aims between the two requirements, which would bring together many of the same stakeholders, FDA has combined the FDASIA and PDUFA requirements and agreements. FDA's first step toward meeting these responsibilities was to hold a three-day meeting from January 6 - 8, 2014, during which Agency staff could discuss issues with, and seek input from, various stakeholders. The first day focused on the challenges involved in the development of drugs and biological products to treat rare diseases. The next two days focused on developing drugs, biological products, and devices specifically for children affected by rare diseases.

The meeting was well attended, with an average of 400 participants per day (in-person and by webcast) and included individuals from academic, clinical, and treating communities; patients and advocacy groups; industry; and governmental agencies. Following the meeting, FDA received 14 comments to the post-meeting docket that mostly echoed the discussion and suggestions expressed by panelists and other participants during the meetings.

Continuing the response to the laws' specific requirements and FDA's commitment under PDUFA, this report includes input from the public and FDA and discusses the many complex issues involved in medical product development for people with rare diseases. Following a brief overview of both legislative and FDA efforts over the years to foster development of therapies for these patients, the report summarizes the three days of the public meeting and presents FDA's strategic plan for accelerating the development of the urgently needed therapies for pediatric rare diseases.

Public Meeting: Issues Discussed

A variety of issues were raised and discussed during the three-day meeting, including the following:

- The need for more comprehensive information about the natural history of most rare diseases;
- The importance of public-private, public-public (interagency and intergovernmental) and international partnerships in providing resources and facilitating data collection;
- Recommendations for greater involvement and a more active role of patients and caregivers in therapeutic product development;
- The invaluable contribution of advocacy groups in the development process to educate and recruit patients, and to assist with endpoint selection;
- The concept that patients' and families' willingness to accept risk for participation in clinical trials, and for adopting new therapies, may be greater for those affected by serious and life-threatening rare diseases;
- The challenges of trial design for the study of small, heterogeneous populations, so typical of many rare diseases;
- Methods to overcome the challenges of trial design, such as flexible drug development programs, adaptive trial designs, enrichment strategies, and master protocols;
- Endpoint development and acceptance for use in registration trials (e.g., patient reported outcomes and surrogates); and
- The ways in which benefit–risk assessments guide regulatory decision making.

A number of issues voiced were outside of FDA's jurisdiction, including, considerations of statutory changes; issues dealing with reimbursements; and the governance and management of patient registries.

FDA emphasized the importance of sponsors engaging FDA early and often during the development process to help ensure a more efficient and expedient path to approval and marketing.

Strategic Plan: To Accelerate the Development of Rare Disease Therapies for Children

Two cross-agency workgroups (one for drugs and biological products, another for devices) worked to formulate a strategic plan with the goal of identifying strategies "to encourage and accelerate the development of new therapies (drugs, biological products, and devices) for pediatric rare diseases," responding to the FDASIA requirement. Based on what was heard during the meetings and in the accompanying public dockets, along with the workgroup members' knowledge of pediatrics and rare diseases, FDA formulated four objectives under which key strategies are identified. The strategies are specific approaches that will strengthen and enhance some of the many initiatives FDA already has undertaken while addressing the legislative goal.

The following objectives are defined and ordered chronologically based on the product development process. When a strategy fit under more than one objective, it was placed beneath the objective that it was considered to affect most. The four objectives are as follows:

1. Enhance foundational and translational science for pediatric rare diseases;
2. Strengthen communication, collaboration, and partnering for pediatric rare diseases within and outside FDA;
3. Advance the use of regulatory science to aid clinical trial design and performance for pediatric rare diseases; and
4. Enhance FDA's review process for pediatric rare disease products.

The *first objective*, to enhance foundational and translational science for pediatric rare diseases (PRD), encompasses strategies to fill foundational science information gaps, such as fostering the conduct of natural history studies for pediatric rare diseases and identifying unmet pediatric needs in medical device development. Other strategies under this objective include providing advice to sponsors on common issues in rare disease drug development through guidance documents, and expanding and refining the use of computational modeling, which can predict how a device will perform before the first prototype is made.

The *second objective* is to strengthen communication, collaboration, and partnering for PRD within and outside FDA. FDA partners and collaborates with many stakeholders inside and outside the Agency. These relationships include public-public (interagency, intergovernmental, and international) and public-private interactions and partnerships, which are vitally important in overcoming the challenges to the development of products for rare diseases, including PRD. Such challenges are difficult to overcome by most single entities (e.g., pharmaceutical manufacturer, academic institution, or governmental organization) because such entities generally do not have sufficient resources or expertise to independently develop products to treat PRD efficiently. Additionally, FDA maintains international collaborations can to enable the exchange of information on development, safety, and effectiveness in the globalized pharmaceutical market, and intra-agency collaborations to help to coordinate PRD issues across FDA. Continuing to foster relationships with all stakeholders is critical in meeting this objective.

Objective three is to advance the use of regulatory science to aid clinical trial design and performance for PRD. Regulatory science is the science of developing new tools, standards, and approaches to assess the safety, efficacy, quality, and performance of FDA-regulated products. The aspects of regulatory science that make up the strategies under this third objective are geared toward clinical trial design and performance. Strategies include facilitating increased knowledge of biomarkers and clinical outcome assessments useful for PRD, encouraging the early engagement of product developers with the Center for Drug Evaluation and Research (CDER) Study Endpoints team in instrument development, and the use of web-based resources for education and for navigating regulatory processes. Additionally, development of FDA guidance documents relevant to PRD will also aid in efficiently executed product development for PRD. Four separate guidance documents that contain pediatric-specific information are currently under development. In addition to guidance development, FDA is also developing specific training programs for pediatric clinical investigators. Furthermore, use of modeling and simulation approaches to inform clinical trials of potential products to treat PRD is actively being explored. Finally, strategies to meet this objective for medical devices include further development of the expedited approval pathway for medical devices intended to treat unmet medical needs for life-threatening or irreversibly debilitating diseases or conditions, and analyzing data for approved medical devices to explore the feasibility of shifting certain premarket data requirements for devices to the postmarket setting in appropriate cases.

Objective four involves strategies to enhance FDA's review process for PRD products. Strategies include gaining a better perspective of patients' and caregivers' preferences and what's important to them to more formally incorporate this information into PRD product development. In addition, FDA plans to implement a benefit–risk framework in the review of marketing applications for new drug and biological products, including such applications for PRD. A structured approach to benefit-risk assessment in the review process will enable better communication of the reasoning behind regulatory decisions and ensure, on a more consistent basis, that these decisions are made in an established context that includes an understanding of the severity of the treated condition and the adequacy of available therapies. Other strategies include the continued implementation of the Rare Pediatric Disease Priority Review Voucher Program which is intended to promote the development of products for the treatment of PRD. In addition to the numerous guidance documents under development as described above, FDA is planning to issue a draft guidance document on the Rare Pediatric Disease Priority Review Voucher Program. This guidance document will provide sponsors with the Agency's current thinking on how to facilitate the use of this new provision. Furthermore, the Agency is continuing to provide education and annual reviewer training for rare disease and PRD that will help promote consistency of scientific and regulatory approaches for PRD and rare disease product applications across FDA review teams. Finally, FDA is exploring the potential for further innovation in data analysis for small population clinical trials, including trials for PRD, which may help to overcome some of the challenges related to the interpretability of small clinical trials.

In summary, FDA's strategic plan outlines key objectives and specific strategies for encouraging and accelerating development of new therapies for PRD. By enhancing and strengthening the many ongoing FDA initiatives that affect all aspects of the development process, FDA can foster innovation in this area of special need.

1. INTRODUCTION

1.1. Background

This report responds to specific statutory requirements in the Food and Drug Administration Safety and Innovation Act (FDASIA)[4] and agreements in the Prescription Drug User Fee Act (PDUFA) Reauthorization Performance Goals and Procedures Fiscal Years 2013 through FY 2017, intended to respond to the challenges of developing drugs and biological products for rare diseases and therapies and diagnostics for pediatric rare diseases (PRD) patients. The report provides a summary of the three day public meeting held by the Food and Drug Administration (FDA or Agency) to discuss the development of these therapies and diagnostics (hereafter "therapies"), discusses public and Agency input related to the development of these therapies and sets forth the FDA's strategic plan for accelerating development of PRD therapies.

1.2. Challenges in Developing Therapies for Rare Diseases and PRD

The definition of a *rare disease* in the 1984 amendments[5] of the Orphan Drug Act[6] (ODA) includes a disease that affects fewer than 200,000 people in the United States.[7] Yet, the National Institutes of Health (NIH) reports that nearly 7,000 rare diseases affect more than 25 million Americans and their families.[8] Approximately 80% of rare diseases are genetic in origin,[9] and about half of all rare diseases affect children[10].

Developing safe and effective products to treat rare diseases can be very challenging. One key reason is that the numbers of patients affected by any individual disease is small, making the study of therapies in such a population difficult. Because many rare diseases exhibit a number of variations or sub-types, there are even smaller numbers of patients with each sub-type, and patients with the individual disease may have highly diverse clinical manifestations and disease progression. Furthermore, there is often a paucity of clinical investigators and a limited number of specialized treatment centers knowledgeable about any given rare disease. The clinical course of any given disease is often not well understood because of the rarity, which leads to difficulty in designing and conducting clinical trials (e.g., identification and selection of meaningful endpoints, such as biomarkers or clinical outcome assessment (COA) measures to assess the effects of the intervention).

For a number of reasons, developing drugs, biological products, and devices (medical products)[11] for pediatric[12] rare diseases is even more challenging. Because a majority of rare diseases are genetic in origin,[13] they significantly affect the pediatric population. Yet, as a group, children comprise a smaller percentage of the overall population, making it especially difficult to recruit adequate numbers of patients. Often, even though there may be evidence of safety and effectiveness in adults, there is a lack of sufficient information about medical product safety and effectiveness in pediatric populations. A medical product undergoing development must take these issues into account, for all the various age ranges. Additional considerations include the ethical concerns related to clinical testing in children and the need to test in different pediatric sub-groups (e.g., age, maturation of organ function). Last but not least, deficiencies in the pediatric clinical research infrastructure (an issue in the development of medical products for rare diseases in general) can be a key challenge to the planning of clinical trials for pediatric patients.[14]

In recognition of these many challenges, Congress has enacted a number of laws over time to stimulate the development and improve the availability of therapies for patients with rare diseases, and for children.

1.3. Legislation Advancing the Development of Therapies for Rare Diseases and Pediatric Populations

In 1983, Congress passed the *ODA* to promote the development of therapies to prevent, treat, and diagnose rare diseases. This legislation, as amended, and as supplemented by other laws, creates a number of incentives, including financial incentives to develop drugs and biological products (hereafter "drugs") for rare diseases. Incentives include tax credits to offset the cost of clinical trials, waiver of marketing application user fees, and potential eligibility to obtain seven years of marketing exclusivity upon approval of the drug. In addition, an Orphan Products Development (OPD) Grants program was established that supports the clinical development of drugs, biological products for rare diseases. Since the enactment of ODA, more than 3,000 products have received orphan drug designation and been eligible to benefit from the associated financial incentives for development, and more than 460 drugs for rare diseases have been developed and approved for marketing. In addition, more than 500 clinical trials have been supported by FDA's OPD Grants program, resulting in more than 50 medical product approvals.

In 1990, the *Safe Medical Devices Act*[15] established the humanitarian device exemption (HDE) pathway to promote the development of medical devices for rare diseases. A medical device that receives designation as a humanitarian use device (HUD)[16] is eligible to enter the market through this pathway. The HDE pathway exempts a HUD from demonstrating effectiveness if certain criteria are met. The sponsor must demonstrate that the device does not pose an unreasonable or significant risk of illness or injury and that the probable benefit to health outweighs the risk of injury or illness from its use. Since the start of the program, more than 200 products have been designated as a HUD, and 59 have been approved for use in very rare diseases and conditions (hereafter "diseases").[17,18]

In 2002, the *Best Pharmaceuticals for Children Act (BPCA)*[19] was enacted. BPCA provides incentives for sponsors to conduct FDA-requested pediatric studies by granting an additional six months to any existing marketing exclusivity.[20] In 2003, the *Pediatric Research Equity Act (PREA)*[21] gave FDA the authority to require sponsors to submit an assessment of the safety and effectiveness of a drug for the claimed indications in all relevant pediatric subpopulations as part of certain New Drug Applications (NDA), Biologic License Applications (BLA) and supplement applications. In certain cases, PREA allows for deferrals and waivers. Additionally, PREA exempts orphan designated products. Prior to the implementation of these laws, over 80% of drugs contained no pediatric information. Since the implementation of these laws more pediatric trials have been conducted than in the 50 years preceding[22] and 500 labeling changes have been made to incorporate pediatric-specific information, which provides doctors with important information about correct dosage, safety and effectiveness in children.

In 2007, to promote the development of medical devices in the pediatric population, the *Pediatric Medical Device Safety and Improvement Act (PMDSIA)*[23], part of the Food and Drug Administration Amendments Act of 2007 (FDAAA), authorized HUDs to be marketed for a profit when the devices are labeled for pediatric use. In addition, it permitted the extrapolation of adult effectiveness data to support use in a pediatric population. This legislation also created the Pediatric Device Consortia (PDC) Grant Program, which funds various non-profit pediatric device consortia. These consortia make up a network of advisory resources from multiple disciplines to help advance the development of medical devices for use in children. The consortia have assisted with more than 325 pediatric device projects, most of which have been in the early phases of development.

In 2012, *FDASIA* permanently reauthorized BPCA and PREA. In addition, FDASIA created the Rare Pediatric Disease Priority Review Voucher (PRV) program to encourage the development of drugs for PRD. Under this program, the sponsor of a drug for a *rare pediatric disease* may be eligible to receive a PRV upon approval of the drug for that rare pediatric disease, if the criteria of the FDASIA provision are met. The voucher can be redeemed for priority review of another drug application that would not otherwise be eligible for priority review. FDASIA also reauthorized the OPD Grant Program, the PDC Grant program and *PDUFA.* As described later in this report, FDASIA and PDUFA have prompted additional measures to help address the challenges of PRD medical product development, including requiring this report and an FDA strategic plan to advance development of treatments for PRD patients.

1.4. Approaches to Expedite and Accelerate Rare Disease Medical Product Development

Most rare diseases are serious or life-threatening disorders with unmet medical needs.[24] Speeding the development and availability of therapeutics for these serious diseases is important, as they are often the first available treatment or have significant advantages over existing treatments. FDA has developed distinct and successful approaches to making such therapies available as rapidly as possible.

1.4.1. Drugs/Biologics

Priority Review, Accelerated Approval, Fast Track, and Breakthrough Therapy are examples of such approaches for drugs.

FDA first formally articulated its thinking on expediting the availability of promising new drugs in the 1980s, in regulations codified at 21 CFR part 312, subpart E. The subpart E regulations are intended to speed the availability of new drugs to patients with serious conditions (especially when there are no satisfactory alternative therapies) while preserving appropriate standards for safety and effectiveness, such as through early consultation with FDA for sponsors of such products and efficient trial designs.

FDA has a long history of applying the philosophy underlying subpart E to drugs for rare diseases through use of the expedited programs, and additionally recognizes that certain aspects of drug development that are feasible for common diseases may not be feasible for rare diseases and that development challenges are often greater with increasing rarity of the disease.

The expedited programs are summarized below.[25] More detail and information on how to apply for these programs are available in FDA's guidance for industry, Expedited Programs for Serious Conditions – Drugs and Biologics.

- Priority review[26]

An application for a drug may be eligible to receive priority review if it offers a major advance in treatment or provides a treatment when no adequate therapy exists.[27] The goal is to complete priority review marketing application reviews in 6 months, rather than the standard 10 months.

- Accelerated Approval[28]

A drug intended to treat a serious or life-threatening illness and provides meaningful therapeutic benefit over existing treatments may be eligible for accelerated approval. Eligibility is assessed during drug development and marketing application review, usually following discussion with FDA earlier in the drug development process. Through this pathway marketing approval may be granted on the basis of adequate and well-controlled clinical trials that establish an effect of the drug on a surrogate endpoint that is reasonably likely to predict clinical benefit, or on a clinical endpoint other than irreversible morbidity or mortality (IMM). Accelerated Approval requires that the drug be studied further in the postmarket period to verify and describe its clinical benefit or effect on IMM.

- Fast Track[29]

A drug intended to treat a serious disease and fill an unmet medical need may be eligible to receive fast track designation.[30] Designation may be granted on the basis of *preclinical* or *clinical* data. This provision is intended to facilitate development and expedite review. Fast track provides more frequent interactions with FDA (e.g., meetings or written correspondence) during drug development and the use of a rolling review whereby companies can submit completed sections of marketing applications for FDA review, rather than waiting until every section is complete.

- Breakthrough Therapy[31]

Breakthrough Therapy designation may be granted to a drug intended, alone or in combination with other drugs, to treat a serious or life-threatening disease and preliminary *clinical* evidence indicates that the drug may demonstrate substantial improvement over existing therapies. Breakthrough drugs are eligible for all of the Fast Track provisions, intensive FDA guidance on an efficient drug development program, and organizational commitment involving senior managers and experienced cross-disciplinary review staff.

1.4.2. Devices

With regard to medical devices, FDA is proposing an expedited access Premarket Approval (PMA) (EAP) pathway that will be available for medical devices that address unmet medical needs, including those for PRD. This new approach is discussed in more detail in the Strategic Plan.

Already in place for medical devices is the *De Novo* **Classification Process**[32]. This process provides a pathway to manufacturers of novel medical devices, including those for PRD, to reclassify novel devices of low to moderate risk that had automatically been placed in the higher risk Class III after receiving a "not substantially equivalent" determination in response to a premarket notification [510(k)] marketing submission. This alternate pathway limits unnecessary expenditure of FDA and industry resources that could occur if lower risk devices were subject to the premarket approval PMA marketing pathway under section 515 of the Federal Food, Drug, and Cosmetic (FD&C) Act. More detail and information on the *de novo* classification process are provided in the draft guidance document *De Novo Classification Process (Evaluation of Automatic Class III Designation)*.

1.5. FDA's Implementation of Expedited Programs and Flexibility in the Review Process

FDA continues to see new cutting edge, innovative therapies for rare and pediatric diseases, as well as common disease therapies that are repurposed for rare diseases and PRD, and has had success implementing expedited approval pathways for eligible products. In 2013 alone, FDA approved 33 orphan drugs (seven in the Center for Biologics Evaluation and Research [CBER] and 26 in the Center for Drug Evaluation and Research [CDER]). Of the 27 new molecular entities (NMEs) approved in 2013[33]:

- Nine were for orphan products (i.e., rare diseases) (33%);
  - All nine NMEs were approved after the first review cycle
  - Eight were approved first in the United States
- Two used the breakthrough therapy designation pathway;
- Five used fast track; and
- Four used the priority approval pathway.

Under the de novo classification process for medical devices, two diagnostic devices for genetic testing were authorized. These authorizations took advantage of data that had been collecting into a wellcurated database for rare disease mutations for cystic fibrosis, and relied on skilled interpreters for chromosomal copy number changes in developmental diseases, where no single pathogenic change is often seen in multiple patients with similar phenotypes. The precedents set by these recent clearances using the de novo classification process demonstrate FDA's willingness to use the best available database and processes for PRD.

To support these efforts, FDA has made organizational changes, including creating positions in its Centers to facilitate and accelerate the development and approval of medical products to treat rare diseases. Many of these staff also provide scientific and regulatory advice to the sponsors who are working to bring new therapies to market. As highlighted in a recent report by the National Organization for Rare Disorders (NORD)[34], FDA has shown continuing flexibility in the development of products for rare diseases.

FDA's multifaceted and collaborative approach to medical product development and evaluation for rare and pediatric diseases, including expanding support for, and application of, regulatory science to address gaps in knowledge and speed medical product development, is bringing successes and substantial progress. These and future efforts will ensure that FDA continues to serve these special populations, making real differences in their lives.

1.6. Public Meetings and Report(s) under FDASIA and PDUFA Related to Rare Diseases and PRD

1.6.1. Section 510 of FDASIA

Although strides have been made in developing products for rare diseases and for pediatric populations, developing products for PRD continues to be a challenge for the reasons discussed above. To address these challenges, Congress directed FDA to conduct a public meeting and issue a report that includes a strategic plan, focused specifically on PRD. Section 510 of FDASIA enacted on July 9, 2012, specifically required the following:

> **(a) PUBLIC MEETING.**—Not later than 18 months after the date of enactment of the Act, the Secretary shall hold at least one public meeting to discuss ways to encourage and accelerate the development of new therapies for pediatric rare diseases.
> **(b) REPORT.**—Not later than 180 days after the date of the public meeting under section (a), the Secretary shall issue a report that includes a strategic plan for encouraging and accelerating the development of new therapies for treating pediatric rare diseases.

1.6.2. PDUFA Performance Goals

In recognition of the complexities of conducting clinical trials for rare diseases, one of the performance goals that FDA agreed to with industry under Congress' fifth authorization of PDUFA for fiscal years 2013 through 2017, Performance Goal Section IX.E.4., included the following:

> By mid-FY 2014, FDA, through the Rare Disease Program, will **conduct a public meeting** to discuss complex issues in clinical trials for studying drugs for rare diseases, including such questions as endpoint selection, use of surrogate endpoints/Accelerated Approval, and clinical significance of primary endpoints; reasonable safety exposures; assessment of dose selection; and development of patient-reported outcome instruments. Participants in the discussion will include FDA staff, academic and clinical experts, and industry experts. A summary from the meeting will be made available publicly through the FDA website.

1.6.3. Public Meetings ("Workshops")

In response to these two separate but overlapping directives, FDA conducted a three day of public meeting from January 6 - 8, 2014, at FDA in Silver Spring, Maryland. The workshops included input from academic, clinical and treating communities, patients and advocacy groups, industry, and government agencies.

On January 6 & 7, 2014, FDA held a public workshop entitled *Complex Issues in Developing Drug and Biological Products for Rare Diseases,* to discuss complex issues in clinical trials for rare disease drugs and biological products, and to discuss ways to encourage and accelerate the development of new therapies for PRD.

On January 8, 2014, FDA held a separate but related public workshop entitled Complex Issues in Developing Medical Devices for Pediatric Patients Affected by Rare Diseases, to discuss issues associated with medical devices for the diagnosis and treatment of pediatric patients affected by rare diseases.

The public workshops had accompanying public dockets which offered opportunity for interested parties to express their thoughts and provide their input on issues related to therapeutics for rare diseases, including PRD.

1.7. Scope of This Report

This report, which is responsive to both FDASIA section 510(b) and PDUFA V Performance Goal Section IX.E.4, summarizes the outcome of the public meetings and describes a strategic plan for encouraging and accelerating the development of new therapies, including drugs, biological products, and medical devices, for PRD.

The intent of this Strategic Plan is to outline what FDA can reasonably achieve under its authority. Some of the ideas raised at the meetings were outside of FDA's jurisdiction. The ultimate successes stemming from the strategic plan will be the market availability and patient use of safe and effective therapeutics for children with rare diseases. Interim success will be the implementation of the plan outlined in this report.

2. WORKSHOP SUMMARY

2.1. January 6: Public Workshop on Complex Issues in Developing Drug and Biological Products for Rare Diseases

The January 6 workshop focused on four key areas: (1) complex issues in development of clinical and surrogate endpoints, and patient reported outcomes (PROs); (2) complex issues in trial design, conduct, and analysis in rare disease populations; (3) development of foundational, translational, and regulatory science to support rare disease drug development; and (4) safety assessments and dosing considerations in rare disease clinical development programs. A transcript is available at: http://www.fda.gov/downloads/Drugs/NewsEvents/UCM402422.pdf.

Based on these four key areas, the meeting was divided into four sessions, summarized below. Each session summary includes a **background, general overview,** and **technical overview** sections.

2.1.1. Day 1, Session 1: Complex Issues for Trial Design: Endpoints

Chair: Edward M. Cox, M.D., M.P.H., Director, Office of Antimicrobial Products, CDER, FDA

This session can be viewed in its entirety at this link: https://collaboration.fda.gov/p98526rb6kd/.

Background

To effectively study drugs that can be used to treat a disease, researchers must fully understand the disease's natural history. **Natural history** is the term used to describe how a disease would evolve if no treatment was given. However, not all diseases affect every individual in the same way. Therefore, to have a thorough understanding of the natural history of a disease, scientists must observe many patients with the disease over time. In the case of rare diseases, the natural history of a disease is frequently not fully understood because not enough patients with the disease have been observed and studied. Therefore, insufficient knowledge of the natural history of a rare disease is a key impediment in designing and performing clinical trials, and in finding safe and effective treatments. There are thousands of rare diseases, most of which do not currently have adequate natural histories.

When scientists discuss an **"endpoint"** in a clinical trial of a drug, they are referring to the measurement they use to help them determine if the drug is effective. For example, an endpoint may be a measure of how many people who took the drug did not have their disease get significantly worse. A **"surrogate endpoint"** is a measure of an effect of a therapeutic intervention that is known or reasonably likely to indicate the achievement of a clinical endpoint. A specific example of a surrogate endpoint is a measure that shows that a treatment decreased the amount of HIV virus in a patient's blood (viral load), with the thought that this decrease will lead to achieving the clinical endpoint of reducing the risk of dying from AIDS caused by the virus. Measuring endpoints requires a strong understanding of the natural history of a disease and a sound scientific method for effectively measuring its progression. Selecting an appropriate endpoint and then measuring it effectively is often challenging and critically important to the success of any clinical trial, especially one designed to assess the effectiveness of a drug to treat a rare disease.

General Overview

The discussion in this session was focused on the role of information about the natural history of diseases, effects of treatment, and patient benefits in developing endpoints for clinical trials. Panelists explored possible sources of information to characterize the natural history of disease and the effects of treatment. Additionally, panelists considered approaches that could be utilized to facilitate better data collection in natural history registries and endpoint development, and ways in which these efforts might be organized. During this session, it was noted that well-defined endpoints can help facilitate development of new drugs and that unsuccessful clinical trials may have endpoints that were incorrectly identified or measured, thereby potentially losing the benefit of a drug to help treat a condition.

Technical Overview

The panelists discussed organization of natural history studies and disease registries, and emphasized the importance of standardization, transparency, and compatibility of data collection among multiple database holders. The discussants supported the need to modernize the current approaches to data collection and to start developing "second generation" natural history registries that would incorporate data into centralized global repositories. To this end, issues with data sharing, data de-identification, privacy concerns, challenges with motivating researchers to share data, and intellectual property issues were discussed at length. Panelists also noted the need for collaborative approaches and creation of independent governance structures for such registries. A key theme throughout this discussion was the importance of engaging patients and communities, with a suggested approach of creating public-private partnerships to help facilitate information collection in natural history studies and registries.

The challenges and importance of finding endpoints that are clinically meaningful to patients with rare diseases were also discussed during this session. It was suggested that patient advocacy organizations could be hubs for data collection and could help facilitate development of patient-reported outcomes (PROs) for patients with specific diseases. The panelists discussed the key role patients and caregivers play as research partners to facilitate the development of new therapies, by identifying the meaningful signs and symptoms that can enable the development of endpoints for use in future trials.

The panelists further elaborated on various sources of information that could be used in endpoint development. In addition to input from patients, sources named included published case studies, cross-sectional analyses, and prospective longitudinal natural history studies with information on phenotypic and genotypic characteristics of the disease, available biomarkers, and clinical manifestations. The panelists generally agreed that while cross-sectional and longitudinal natural history studies may be the initial steps for endpoint identification, phase 2 is an appropriate stage in drug development programs at which endpoints could be tested. Caution should be exercised in rare disease development programs in which characteristics of patients enrolled in the interventional trials differ from those of patients enrolled in natural history studies. To this end, bypassing phase 2 trials to shorten the development time and proceeding to phase 3 trials without sufficient endpoint characterization may undermine the ability to conduct successful efficacy trials.

2.1.2. Day1, Session 2: Complex Issues for Trial Design: Study Design, Conduct and Analysis

Chair: Ellis F. Unger, M.D., Director, Office of Drug Evaluation-I, Office of New Drugs (OND), CDER, FDA

This session can be viewed in its entirety at this link: https://collaboration.fda.gov/p3vnvfjbncp/

Background

As was noted by many workshop participants, the greatest challenge in designing and interpreting clinical trials in rare diseases is the **small numbers of patients** available for clinical studies. Such small numbers of patients, if studied using conventional study design, are often not sufficient to generate enough data to establish the safety and effectiveness of the drug. Compounding that challenge is the fact that the few patients who are available for study may exhibit signs of the disease in different ways or react to medications intended to treat their condition in different ways. These differences are often referred to as **"heterogeneity."**

General Overview

This session was focused on discussion of alternative clinical trial designs intended to overcome the limitations of small numbers of patients and patient heterogeneity. With a scarcity of patients who have rare diseases available for any given study, it is critical to consider efficient designs and methods enabling the conduct of studies with small numbers of patients. Such methods include various crossover designs, use of historical control studies and enrichment strategies, where appropriate.

Enrichment strategies are used in clinical trials to increase the likelihood that a drug being studied will show the effect of the treatment. FDA has recently issued a draft guidance document titled, *Guidance for Industry on Enrichment Strategies.*

During this session, it was noted that FDA is not risk-averse when it comes to the study of drugs that can potentially treat a rare disease. Many drugs being tested to treat rare diseases may be the only therapeutic option available to the patients with a given condition. Because rare diseases are often serious, debilitating, and fatal, there is general recognition that FDA, patients and physicians are willing to accept greater risk or side effects from drugs that treat rare serious or life-threatening diseases than for drugs that treat non-serious diseases. With increased risk tolerance and acceptance, adequate informed consent for trial participation, and transparent drug labeling reflective of the effects of the drug and its safety profile are critically important.

The session participants discussed the usefulness of patient-specific "chief complaint" endpoints, where patients are asked "What are the one or two things that bother you the most?" This question stimulated much discussion. There was significant agreement among panelists that the approach, essentially representative of asking patients to help define potential future trial endpoints, is not commonly used and should be further encouraged in rare disease development programs.

Technical Overview

The panelists discussed the pros and cons of specific methodologies of various trial designs, including randomized withdrawal design, various crossover designs, "N of 1" design with repeat measurements of individual responses, use of historical control data, and enrichment strategies. Each of these designs has a number of limitations and should be chosen within the context of measured effects in appropriate rare disease settings.

Enrichment strategies, including identification of patient subpopulations based on genetic or susceptibility testing, were discussed in the context of rare disease populations. It was noted that while enrichment designs include patients who would be more likely to respond to therapy, the testing of a product in a carefully chosen subset of patients should be considered in the context of future labeling and the likelihood for postmarketing use of the drug by all patients with the rare condition. Several panelists noted that trial duration should be of appropriate length for chronic irreversible conditions. Handling of missing data in small size trials often presents a challenge and may become an impediment to successful trial conduct and analysis. The trials in rare diseases should therefore, be carefully designed to balance sufficient patient participation and appropriate trial duration.

It was noted that in rare disease development programs, an "all inclusive" strategy may be worthy of consideration. In parallel with ongoing trials, companion protocols and expanded access programs should be considered for patients who do not qualify for, or are unable to participate in, the trial but who may benefit from use of investigational treatment.

The aspect of risk tolerance and acceptance was discussed from the perspective of patients, physicians, and regulators. It was pointed out that FDA is not risk averse, acknowledges that patients and physicians are willing to accept greater risks when dealing with serious diseases, and promotes transparency in informing patients and healthcare providers about risks, toxicities and limitations of investigational products through informed consent and appropriate product labeling once the product is approved.

The topic of statistical analysis in small trials in rare populations was briefly discussed by the panelists and then raised again with a question from the audience. It was opined that alternatively to the widely employed statistical methodologies, Bayesian statistics and use of probability modeling may constitute other options to consider in rare disease trial designs, where appropriate in specific disease settings.

2.1.3. Day 1, Session 3: Foundational Science

Chair: Marc K. Walton, M.D., Ph.D., Associate Director, Office of Translational Sciences, CDER, FDA This session can be viewed in its entirety at this link: https://collaboration.fda.gov/p7n2jt4epvb/

Background

Foundational science is science of any type that *enables* successful drug development, but is not the scientific work that is the actual drug development. In other words, foundational science provides the *background* science that supports clinical trials for the study of potential therapies to treat rare diseases. Collection and analysis of information about **natural history** of a rare disease is a key foundational science in the study of rare diseases (see summary of Session 1 for a description of the term, natural history), because it enables understanding of the complex disease mechanisms and clinical manifestations. Another form of foundational science used to aid drug development is the use of **animal models** of rare diseases. By studying rare diseases in animals, scientists can learn more about the rare disease while reducing risk to people, and can study aspects of the disease unable to be studied in people. One aspect of foundational science used to support clinical trials is the development and use of **biomarkers**. This term refers to biological (e.g., blood tests) measurements, physical signs (e.g., blood pressure), or radiologic testing, taken to assess the activity of a disease or the effect of a drug.

General Overview

This session focused on the discussion of the role of natural history knowledge in rare disease drug development and the ways to obtain this knowledge. The importance of animal models of a disease in drug development, as well as their limitations, were highlighted and discussed. The session participants discussed where in the process of drug discovery biomarkers could play a role and what the impact of using biomarkers in development programs would be. The panelists further explored where resources could be found to support the advancement of natural history studies, animal models, and biomarkers to further facilitate the development of therapies for rare diseases.

Technical Overview

In addition to the discussion of natural history studies during Session 1, the panelists discussed the constraints and benefits of longitudinal studies, and opportunities to develop biorepositories within natural history studies. One approach suggested and echoed by several discussants was that of a mixed model for collecting data and utilizing available tools in natural history studies to include: (1) data collection in study centers during patients visits, (2) remote data collection through instruments completed by patients and caregivers from home, and (3) utilization of electronic data collection from existing electronic medical records through their integration with natural history data collections.

The role of animal models was recognized as useful in both understanding the disease mechanisms and in obtaining information about the toxicological effects of drugs. With regard to the disease mechanisms, it was noted that focusing on the primary physiology of a disease may yield more benefit from animal models than trying to align clinical responses across different species. The panelists agreed on the potential usefulness of animal models in establishing proof-of-concept for new drugs, but also noted that it is important to understand where differences between species create information that cannot be relied upon, because observations in humans with a rare disease may differ from those in animal models. One approach mentioned during the session suggested using experiments with targeted use of patients' cell lines for scientific bridging between animal studies and human studies. The utility of comparative animal modeling was discussed, and the distinction between the animal models of naturally occurring disease and artificial models (e.g., laboratory genetic knock out models) was emphasized as a factor that should be considered when obtaining data about disease pathogenesis.

There was a general agreement that animal studies are necessary for understanding the toxicological effects of new drugs and, in some cases, are useful in determining appropriate dose finding. Since there is often urgency to advance research to treat serious disorders, the panelists discussed the difficult question of how much time should be spent on animal studies and when there sufficient information to move to human studies. In general, it was noted that the amount of toxicological data needed in each program remains largely dependent on the effects and qualities of the product and the human experience in similar drug classes which would be expected to vary among drug programs.

FDA guidance documents that describe standard toxicological studies expected in development programs are available.

The discussion relating to biomarkers focused largely on early phase trials and included deliberations about scientific and logistical approaches to biomarker qualification, and the importance of understanding the purpose and utility of a biomarker within a given development program (e.g., prognostic, predictive, pharmacokinetic/pharmacodynamics [PK/PD] measures, etc.). The panelists recognized the prolonged time that it takes to develop and qualify biomarkers, as well as the need to find other approaches and alternative modeling to shorten the qualification time. In certain cases, a biomarker may provide value and precision in measurement, for example, in situations where measuring a clinical outcome is not feasible, such as when it would take many years to measure. In early developmental stages for new therapies, understanding the dynamics of a biomarker's change is helpful in understanding disease pathophysiology and when additional information is needed, such as for decisions of dose selection. One panel discussant pointed out that including biomarkers in longitudinal natural history studies can be valuable for development of future therapies.

When discussing the resources available to support foundational science, it was pointed out that many traditional sources of research funding, such as investigators' grant programs, are financially strained. Several panelists noted that patient advocacy organizations have been, and remain a strong support for the advancement of foundational sciences. It was also suggested that mixed funding from various sources, including federal and corporate organizations, often need to be utilized to provide more resilience and consistency for the support of foundational science projects. The lack of sufficient funding was identified as an important gap.

2.1.4. Day 1, Session 4: Safety and Dosing

Chair: Mwango Kashoki, M.D., Associate Director for Safety, OND CDER, FDA

This session can be viewed in its entirety at this link: https://collaboration.fda.gov/p51uf9yw2fh

Background

In addition to assessing a drug's *efficacy* during a clinical trial, it is also critical to assess a drug's *safety* (i.e., adverse drug reactions). As with other challenges in clinical trials for drugs intended to treat rare diseases, the small number of patients involved in trials also affects researchers' and drug developers' ability to assess safety. An important aspect of assessing the safety of a drug during clinical trials is the **selection of an appropriate dose to be tested**; too low a dose may lead to a failed study in which no benefit of the drug could be detected, but too high a dose could also lead to a failed study because the drug is shown to cause excessive or unacceptable adverse side effects. Researchers and drug developers must also consider what is a reasonable safety exposure (i.e., the number of patients, for what period of time, and route of administration) in order to assess the frequency, magnitude and severity of a drug's adverse effects.

Because clinical trials for rare disease therapies are often too small to definitively ascertain a drug's complete safety profile (e.g., uncommon adverse drug reactions), it is important and often necessary to continue to assess the drug's safety after it has been approved and is being used in a larger patient population (**pharmacovigilance**). Effective pharmacovigilance can help detect additional safety issues that researchers and drug developers were unable to detect during the premarketing period.

Patient registries are another tool used to monitor outcomes in patients after a clinical trial. Patient registries allow for long-term follow-up of patients and can foster enduring relationships among patients with rare diseases, their caregivers, health care providers, and drug developers.

For certain drugs, FDA may require implementation of a set of measures and rules that healthcare providers and patients can follow to ensure safe use of these drugs. Such a set of safety measures and rules is referred to as **Risk Evaluation and Mitigation Strategy (REMS)**. A **REMS** program may be required for a drug in its postmarketing period to ensure that the benefits of the drug outweigh its risks. **REMS with Elements to Assure Safe Use (ETASU)** can be implemented in settings where access to a drug is conditioned, for example, upon certain qualifications of healthcare providers and appropriate informing of patients about safe use of the drug. When considering a REMS program with ETASU for a rare disease drug, the potential effects of limited access should be carefully considered.

General Overview

This session explored approaches to safety assessments of drugs intended to treat rare diseases in both premarketing development and the postmarketing period. Issues discussed included the small size of the clinical trials, challenges in determining the adequate drug exposure (what dose(s) to study and what duration of exposure to assess), and determination of an appropriate sized safety database. The panelists also discussed approaches to safety assessments in determining appropriate dosing regimens for drugs. The panelists explored enhanced pharmacovigilance strategies for drugs to treat rare diseases and innovative ways to utilize postmarketing patient registries to collect additional drug safety data. Some panelists noted that by entering into the field of drug development for a rare disease, sponsors are essentially beginning or continuing work in the area of establishing the disease's natural history, and characterizing the disease prevalence. This work is fostering long-term relationships and commitments between drug developers, researchers, and patients with rare conditions, which is necessary to move science forward and to generate effective therapies. The panelists also considered when the use of registries and REMS programs is appropriate and, if so, how researchers and health care providers can maximize their benefits.

Technical Overview

The panelists discussed the challenges of establishing a one-size-fits-all standard of a premarketing safety database, and with assessing duration of exposure to a drug in rare disease development programs. Several discussants opined that the size of the safety database is often informed by the estimated size of the population with a rare condition (i.e., disease prevalence), and suggested that following patients for a longer period of time could, in some cases, compensate for the smaller sizes of the clinical trial populations. Others suggested that safety exposure should mirror how the drug will be used in clinical practice after approval. There was general agreement that feasibility issues (e.g., ability to adequately recruit patients for enrollment into a trial) also impact the size of a clinical program. It was suggested that rather than always attempting to increase the numbers of patients in clinical trials, there should be efforts to improve methods of and approaches to safety data collection, with the goal to decrease redundancy and increase value of the collected data. To this end, leveraging data from animal models and natural history studies may facilitate understanding of the expected drug effects and the disease-related health outcomes, to enable finding a more targeted approach to adverse event collection and assessment.

With regard to dose selection, the panelists suggested that the clinical trials should assess the safety of a range of doses, rather than focusing on a single dose. It was agreed that the design of the trial can impact the evaluation of drug safety, and there were suggestions that novel or different methods be used to explore the safety of doses (e.g., adaptive dose finding, use of biomarkers in dose finding and dose response). One discussant pointed out that in rare disease development programs, sponsors sometimes have to conduct first-in-human studies in patients with the disease, instead of in healthy volunteers (e.g., enzyme replacement therapies). Discussion about risk tolerance centered on patient's and health care provider's risk tolerance. It was generally agreed upon that risk tolerance varies among individual patients and caregivers, and across patient populations, with different levels of risk acceptance in different diseases. Risk tolerance would also be expected to change as more treatments become available for a particular condition. It was pointed out that risk tolerance is built through education about the disease and the effects of available and new therapies. Health care providers can impact and inform patients' and caregivers' risk tolerance; providers are frequently asked to give their assessments of the risks and benefits of a drug. The panelists suggested that there be a formal framework for assessing and balancing benefit-risk assessments of drugs used to treat rare diseases.

With regard to longitudinal safety data collection, it was mentioned that obtaining long-term safety data can be achieved through extensions of established clinical trials or through post-marketing studies, to enable better understanding of long-term effects of drugs, particularly drugs approved for chronic use. The challenges of long-term follow-up were also discussed, including the difficulties in maintaining longterm relationships with international clinical trial participants, the potential for patients' "study fatigue," and patients' desire to switch to a newly emerging and promising therapy.

The panelists found that pharmacovigilance of drugs used to treat rare diseases is not necessarily different from that for drugs used to treat common diseases. The pharmacovigilance strategies employed will, for both rare and common disease drugs, depend on such factors as the nature of the product, the adverse events of concern, and the extent of safety data already available.

The role of REMS programs in ensuring that the benefits outweigh the risks for patients with rare diseases was discussed. The panelists considered when a REMS with ETASU would be appropriate for a drug intended to treat a rare disease. While differing opinions were expressed by the panelists, it was generally recognized that although a REMS with ETASU program may create an additional burden for clinicians and patients, it may also be the only practical means to ensure patients' access to drugs that would otherwise not be considered safe for use in clinical practice. The discussion further included assessments of opportunities and strategies for balancing REMS issues of improving patients' access to medicines and decreasing the burden of implementation of safety measures. It was noted that when considering postmarketing safety efforts, it is important to keep in mind the seriousness of the conditions being treated and the absence of alternative therapies to treat them. To this end, the anticipated product's benefit, as well as the level of risk tolerance, would influence decisions about design and implementation of REMS programs.

2.2. January 7: Public Workshop on Encouraging and Accelerating Development of New Drugs and Biologics for PRD

The January 7 workshop set out to explore (1) pediatric clinical trial development, including pediatric clinical networks, (2) pediatric risk assessment, (3) oncology related issues, and, (4), gene therapy related issues. The meeting was divided into four sessions, reflecting the four areas mentioned above. The structure for Day 2 consisted of no formal presentations; rather there was informal dialogue with exchange of ideas. The summaries below aim to reflect those discussions. A transcript is available at: http://www.fda.gov/downloads/Drugs/NewsEvents/UCM402423.pdf.

2.2.1. Day 2, Session 1: Networks and Collaborations in Support of Pediatric Clinical Trials

Chair: Anne Zajicek, M.D., Pharm.D., Chief, Obstetric and Pediatric Pharmacology and Therapeutics Branch, Eunice Kennedy Shriver National Institute of Child Health and Human Development (NICHD) This session can be viewed in its entirety at: https://collaboration.fda.gov/p8ubdu5c8hp/.

Background

A **pediatric clinical trial network** is an association of independent clinical research sites located throughout the U.S., and sometimes also in other countries, that cooperate in designing and conducting pediatric clinical trials to improve health care for pediatric patients. In rare diseases, where patient numbers are limited, conducting successful clinical trials can be challenging. One of the benefits offered by pediatric clinical trial networks is the ability to overcome the challenge of small patient numbers for the conduct of successful clinical trials. NIH has expanded the formation of pediatric trial networks to accommodate pediatric studies based on written requests referred to NIH by FDA under BPCA.

General Overview

The panelists in this session shared a wide range of experiences forming, operating and collaborating with successful pediatric clinical trial networks. They shared their views on elements, both good and bad, of clinical trial networks for pediatric research, including (1) adequate management infrastructure, (2) appropriate study protocol with achievable endpoints, (3) clinical investigator capability to enroll patients and perform clinical trials, (4) adequate investigational product, (5) patient involvement, and, (6) an effective data monitoring committee. Panelists also addressed the role of advocacy groups in developing effective pediatric clinical trials networks, as well as ways in which networks help to accelerate pivotal clinical trials of new therapies (e.g., through the use of biomarkers and other surrogate endpoints).

Technical Overview

The focus of the session was on the need for networks to perform the rare disease research necessary for drug or device approvals. Although each panel members' comments highlighted the wide variation in the way pediatric clinical trials networks are structured and operated, many common issues were raised.

First, the important role patient advocates play in the development of research agendas, protocols, and clinically meaningful outcome measures was stressed, as well as their role in addressing the ongoing challenge of patient enrollment in clinical trials. Second, the need for both longitudinal natural history registries and patient contact registries was acknowledged, and that organization, data access and control, and funding of these registries are issues that need to be considered. Third, the importance of having foundational research, gaining agreement with regulatory bodies on pre-defined, validated endpoints, and clinician training to perform clinical research was emphasized. It was agreed upon that when developing pediatric trial endpoints, outcome measures that are important to children must be taken into consideration. The importance for data to be usable by U.S., as well as other regulatory bodies was also discussed, and the panelists agreed that research should be performed in accordance with both U.S. and international standards, and noted that harmonization of processes can facilitate networks' ability to share information and collaborate.

2.2.2. Day 2, Session 2: Tolerating Risk and Uncertainty in Pediatric Clinical Trials

Chair: Robert "Skip" Nelson, M.D., Ph.D., Deputy Director and Senior Pediatric Ethicist, Office of Pediatric Therapeutics (OPT), FDA

This session can be viewed in its entirety at: https://collaboration.fda.gov/p13paf7d2mb/

General Overview

The focus of this session was to discuss how to decide whether sufficient risk-benefit data exists to support giving an experimental product to a child with a life-threatening disease. This decision involves a consideration of the desired clinical benefit, the risks one would be willing to tolerate in hopes of achieving that benefit, and the uncertainty surrounding both in a clinical trial setting. Parents from both the panel and the audience agreed that the hope of delaying disease progression in order to give their child a more fulfilling childhood experience was beneficial. The uncertainty of the risk of an experimental intervention in order to delay disease progression was contrasted with the certainty of progressive deterioration and death. There was consensus that this complex decision must be made collaboratively among all stakeholders and that given the certainty of the life-threatening and progressive nature of many PRD, a greater amount of risk and uncertainty in the hopes of halting an otherwise inevitable disease progression may be tolerable.

Technical Overview

An important decision that is made when developing products for the treatment of rare pediatric diseases is whether there are sufficient data to support giving an experimental product to a child. This decision becomes more critical in first-in-human testing of a product for rare and life-threatening diseases with no known treatments. The panelists focused on three concepts that help to inform this decision: (1) the desired clinical benefit; (2) the probability and nature of the harms (i.e., risks) that may be acceptable to attain those benefits; and (3) the amount of uncertainty about each that is tolerable.

The data needed to support investigational use of a product in children should establish the possibility that each child may benefit clinically from the product. While studies in adults are often used for this purpose, adult data may be unobtainable or uninformative if the disease occurs only in children. In such cases, nonclinical (i.e., animal) disease models must be used. However, relevant animal models may also be unavailable or poorly informative. It may also be scientifically uninformative and/or unethical to ask healthy human adults to volunteer for early phase studies to determine a maximum tolerated dose and/or to obtain preliminary safety data. Therefore, little may be known about the potential benefits and risks of an experimental product prior to the first child's enrollment. Given these uncertainties, it is important for FDA and sponsors to partner early in the product development process and reach agreement on potential paths forward.

The panelists agreed that when considering whether the risks of an experimental product are either "reasonable" or "justified," both the type of harm that the product may cause, and likelihood that the harm may occur should be considered. There was consensus that patients' and families' attitudes about benefit-risk should be solicited as part of the process, but it was acknowledged that these attitudes may change over time, with disease progression. Patient advocates noted that stabilization may be seen as a reasonable benefit, as opposed to the ideal of a cure, and that even the risks for certain harms may be acceptable given the potential for slowed progression of the disease.

There was consensus among all panelists that each stakeholder in the development of new therapies for PRD brings an important perspective to the decision of evaluating whether sufficient data exists to support giving an experimental product to a child. An investigator and/or sponsor must review the data and decide whether to initiate a clinical trial. A regulator must decide whether the data are sufficient to allow a clinical trial to proceed. A parent must decide whether to enroll his or her child in a clinical trial. Ultimately the decision is a collaborative effort.

2.2.3. Day 2, Session 3: Pediatric Oncology

Chair: Gregory Reaman, M.D., Associate Director of Oncology Sciences, Office of Hematology and Oncology Products, CDER, FDA; Professor of Pediatrics, the George Washington University School of Medicine and Health Sciences

This session can be viewed in its entirety at: https://collaboration. fda.gov/p3d8ayp2by5/.

Background

Cancer is the most common disease cause of pediatric death. While pediatric oncology has been part of a paradigm in which treatment efforts have enjoyed a strong level of success in improving outcomes for children with cancer, there remain a great many cancers for which there are no therapies. In the setting of life-threatening diseases, including cancer, the acceptable level of risk of toxicity from a new therapeutic product is likely to be considerably greater than that for many other new drug products. Moreover, the benefit of a new therapy for children with cancer focuses on optimizing chances for cure, and reducing risk of acute and delayed treatment-related toxicities.

General Overview

This session focused on the assessments of risk, assessment tools, and international regulatory issues.

There was agreement that benefit-risk assessment in deciding whether to initiate investigational use of a product should involve broad stakeholder input and that clinical trials should incorporate endpoints using outcome assessments (e.g., symptom improvement and functional performance), in addition to overall survival. There was consensus on the need to further construct and validate clinical outcome assessment tools for prospective use in pediatric clinical trials. It was noted that a sponsor's concerns about individual patient risk may be greater than the actual concerns held by parents and investigators, and that there should be an increased effort to educate sponsors on patients' perspectives. There was general agreement that since product development has become a global enterprise, increased communication between and among sponsors and regulators will facilitate a more efficient overall process.

Technical Overview

The panel seemed to agree that given the bleak life expectancy of relapsed and refractory patients, the potential for any possible benefit should outweigh individual patient risks. There was agreement that the current paradigm for evaluating investigational drugs be expanded to include indications for relapsed patients when the likelihood of cure is extremely low. It was also agreed that if compelling pre-clinical evidence and biologic rationale exists for the investigational use of a specific product, it should be acceptable for first-in-human studies to begin in children. Again, such decisions should be based on broad stakeholder input.

The widely accepted and preferred endpoint for pivotal trials of new products to treat pediatric cancers is overall survival, or a surrogate endpoint which is likely to predict an overall survival benefit. The timelines required for these trials frequently exceed 5-7 years. Consideration of intermediate endpoints or surrogates may facilitate drug development timelines for promising new products for childhood cancers. There was broad agreement that efforts to incorporate the use of outcome assessment measures related to symptoms and functionality be greatly expanded. The panel agreed that patient input was important in developing relevant PROs, designing and testing instruments for assessment, and in designing studies where such assessments might be used.

Because FDASIA requires earlier submission of pediatric study plans for those sponsors subject to PREA, it was noted that opportunities exist to expedite and facilitate discussions between FDA and industry. It was also acknowledged that early discussions of potential agents at the Pediatric Subcommittee of Oncologic Drugs Advisory Committee meetings may help increase the number and quality of Written Requests[35]. Concerns were raised about situations where novel product development programs are terminated because of failed trials in adult cancers when there is potential for use in pediatric cancers. Developing public-private partnerships and providing broader awareness of incentives through BPCA and the Pediatric Rare Disease Priority Review Voucher Program may help increase industry interest to participate in trials to evaluate these otherwise failed/abandoned drugs.

Pediatric cancer drug development is associated with risk and safety concerns largely related to the risk of acute, persistent, or late toxicity of investigational products in children. The perspective of risk is stakeholder dependent. For example, the risk of potentially eroding good outcomes of current therapy by adding or substituting an investigational agent in the experimental arm of a clinical trial is a concern to investigators and regulatory agencies. The risk of jeopardizing an important drug development plan due to the unanticipated adverse experience in a child may be a concern to sponsors. Inaccurate conclusions related to an individual patient's risk tolerance are a concern to parents and investigators. Increased transparency and opportunities for dialogue are needed.

New cancer drug development is a global enterprise. International regulatory agencies assume responsibility for the evaluation and approval of marketing authorization of new drugs. Pediatric-focused legislation, which provides regulatory authority to these agencies, differs with respect to timelines for submission and extent of proposed pediatric development plans. These procedural differences are reported to be a source of delay in initiating early evaluation of new cancer drug products in children. There was considerable discussion of the Office of Pediatric Therapeutics' Pediatric Cluster calls with European Medicines Agency (EMA) and the Common Commentary process. Although there was agreement that such collaborations were helpful and a means of addressing the unintended consequences of differing pediatric regulatory requirements, there was agreement by investigators and industry that more was needed. Wider announcement to industry of the availability of this mechanism to foster joint discussion and coordinated regulatory review of pediatric development plans was suggested. "Master" or "cloud" protocols where a single protocol could evaluate multiple agents simultaneously or sequentially in the same disease, or across multiple diseases, were also suggested. There was agreement that continued discussions between EMA and FDA were required to better coordinate later stage investigational plans for new drugs. There was also agreement that early transparency in FDA's BPCA Written Request process and negotiations that mirror the level of EMA's Pediatric Investigational Plan process to achieve earlier, and more effective coordination in global development plans, would assist industry and investigators and, most importantly, benefit patients.

2.2.4. Day2, Session 4: Gene Therapy Trials in Pediatric Patients

Chair: Ilan Irony, M.D., Chief, General Medicine Branch, Division of Clinical Evaluation and Pharmacology/Toxicology, Office of Cellular, Tissue and Gene Therapies (OCTGT), CBER, FDA This session can be viewed in its entirety at: https://collaboration.fda.gov/p34q1iktipx/

General Overview

The spectrum of diseases for which gene transfers or therapies (hereafter referred to as gene therapies) may be used is wide-ranging. Since children potentially have many years of life ahead of them, the issue of possible long term permanent effects of gene therapy is critical. These issues include the need to address long-term safety risks for children and the requirement for long-term safety follow-up. This session focused on a discussion of the development of products with uncertainty regarding their longterm benefits and risks.

Technical Overview

Gene therapy may provide the prospect of a cure or substantial amelioration of a condition after a single administration of the product. Patients may also incur gene-therapy related harms, which may be prolonged or which may appear only after a long interval following treatment. For this reason, long term follow-up is critical for gene therapy trials. The decision to participate in trials requiring long term safety follow up is based on the natural history of the disease, the stage of disease, and whether longterm follow-up is prohibitive. This decision is also dependent upon whether other treatment options exist. The size of the safety database necessary for marketing application is based primarily on the severity of the disease and the availability of approved alternative therapies. A number of panelists stated that gene therapy product labels must convey the uncertainty regarding the potential risks, and that long-term follow-up should continue postmarketing, to further define these risks. This same transparency about the known or potential benefits and risks should be reflected in the informed consent process for participation in trials.

There was some discussion related to funding gene therapy product development programs. Panelists suggested establishing alliances between patient advocacy groups and commercial or academic sponsors, and for academic institutions to cost-share international sites. Increasing participation of international sites could also lead to faster enrollment of subjects in trials, greater, more comprehensive registries of specific gene therapies, and overall general expansion of gene therapy registries.

Panelists also discussed the potential risks of triggering an immune response from proteins expressed by gene therapy, which may neutralize the benefit of that gene therapy or cause other adverse effects. They also discussed approaches for dealing with pre-existing immunity against viruses used as vectors for gene therapies.

2.3. Summary of Comments from the Public Docket for Days 1 and 2

Twelve comments were submitted to the public docket. The majority of the comments echoed the discussion and suggestions expressed by panelists and other participants during the first day of the meeting. Additional suggestions included recommendations to conduct disease-specific scientific meetings and to continue collaborative efforts and focused discussions in individual rare disease fields. Other areas of interest that were mentioned included:

- Extrapolation of drug effects to sub-populations within orphan indications;
- Elucidation of patient viewpoints on benefit-risk assessment at early stages of the product development process (e.g., before pre-Investigational New Drug Application (IND) meetings);
- Integration of patient perspectives into the drug development process and regulatory decision-making;
- Finding innovative ways to incentivize the development of new treatments;
- Identification of ways sponsors can engage FDA early in the development process to discuss how to build a more robust pathophysiological map of a rare disease as the basis for designing a clinical development program;
- Inclusion of benefit-risk assessment into the framework for biomarker qualification process;

- Development of quantitative assessments for risk tolerance in rare diseases;
- Development of a scientific framework for utilization of the accelerated approval pathway in rare disease drug development; and
- Finding better or more uniformed ways to define disease burden and treatment impact in rare diseases.

The following topics were suggested for inclusion in future FDA guidance documents:

- Development of a framework on selection of surrogate and intermediate clinical endpoints in rare diseases; addressing possible issues arising with the accelerated approval pathway in rare disease populations;
- PROs in rare disease drug development;
- Reliance on nonclinical data in rare disease drug development;
- Conduct of natural history studies in rare diseases, including data aggregation from different sources and identification of FDA's role in setting standards and achieving interoperability across registries and patient datasets; and
- Dose-finding issues in small populations.

2.4. January 8: Public Workshop – Complex Issues in Developing Medical Devices for Pediatric Patients Affected by Rare Diseases

The January 8 workshop was divided into eight sessions, summarized below.

2.4.1. Day 3, Session 1: What's Happening Clinically
Moderator: Linda Ulrich, M.D., Director, Pediatric Device Consortia Grant Program, Office of Orphan Products Development (OOPD), FDA
This session can be viewed in its entirety at Webcast Part 1. A transcript is available at: http://www.fda.gov/downloads/MedicalDevices/NewsEvents/WorkshopsConferences/UCM403799.pdf.

2.4.1.1. Clinician's View

James Geiger, M.D., Professor of Surgery, Executive Director, Medical Innovation Center, University of Michigan.

General Overview

This presentation by Dr. Geiger, a pediatric surgeon, focused on his clinician's view of key challenges in pediatric surgery, where adult medical devices are often used to operate on children. These tools are often much too large and frequently require surgeons to improvise their techniques. Off-label use of adult medical devices is not optimal in the care of children, especially infants.

Technical Overview

Dr. Geiger pointed out that if products sized and designed for children are not considered in the initial iterations of a device, they continue to be left out as subsequent iterations of a given device are developed. He has many ideas for devices potentially suitable for pediatrics, but bringing these ideas to fruition is fraught with challenges. One of these challenges is the need to have multiple sizes to accommodate various sizes of pediatric patients. There are limitations on manufacturers and hospitals in the number of different sizes of each device they can produce and stock, respectively. Therefore, even when child-sized devices are commercially available, these products might not be physically available when and where needed, due to these practical limitations. Dr. Geiger stated that adverse events from inappropriate use of adult devices in children occur every day and are generally not captured in safety reporting. This is in part, because such adverse events are "accepted" as just being part of practice, and also because available reporting mechanisms are perceived as cumbersome and not always effective.

Dr. Geiger indicated that financial issues related to the relatively smaller pediatric market size compared to adults are a key factor in the lack of surgical tools specifically designed for pediatric use, and that while business generally thinks in terms of the cost to develop a device, thinking beyond to broader societal costs (e.g., lives saved, long-term hospitalizations, and disabilities prevented) is necessary for advancement. He suggested that solutions, while challenging, are possible. Effective partnerships were noted as a means to help solve these problems. Small companies utilizing start-up investments can help develop a device and "de-risk" it for later assumption by larger companies. Dr. Geiger also suggested the possibility of adapting the L3C business model, a hybrid between non-profit and for-profit corporate structures to advance socially beneficial products, to be applied in the development of pediatric medical devices. The NIH-sponsored Pediatric Clinical Trials Network is another possible resource to advance pediatric device development, providing harmonized protocol reviews and approaches to address multiple Institutional Review Boards (IRBs).

2.4.2. Day 3, Session 2: What We're Doing

Moderator: Jacqueline Francis, M.D., Medical Officer, Division of Surgical Devices, Center for Devices and Radiological Health (CDRH), FDA

This session can be viewed in its entirety at Webcast Part 1

2.4.2.1. Pediatric Device Issues Update

Jacqueline Francis, M.D., Medical Officer, Division of Surgical Devices, CDRH, FDA

Background

CDRH is responsible for ensuring the safety and effectiveness of medical devices and eliminating unnecessary human exposure to man-made radiation from medical, occupational and consumer products. The Humanitarian Use Device (HUD)/ Humanitarian Device Exemption (HDE) Program was created as an alternative pathway for getting market approval for medical devices for rare diseases or conditions.

Technical Overview

This presentation focused on programs and initiatives within CDRH aimed at addressing pediatric issues.

Dr. Francis began with an overview of changes to the HDE program under FDASIA, including: (1) expanding the current pediatric profit provision to additional rare diseases, allowing sponsors to profit from devices that are intended to treat or diagnose rare diseases or conditions that either do not occur in pediatrics or that occur in such small numbers that the development of the device for children is not possible or is impracticable, or is unsafe; (2) revising the cap on the annual distribution number (ADN) which is defined as the number of devices reasonably needed to treat, diagnose, or cure a population of 4,000 individuals in the United States per year; and (3) allowing sponsors of devices already approved under an HDE to seek the determination for an exemption from profit prohibition.

Dr. Francis also presented three FDA guidance documents that were either in development or issued as draft guidance. The draft guidance titled *Providing*

Information about Pediatric Uses of Medical Devices describes how sponsors compile and submit readily available pediatric use information. The draft guidance titled *Pediatric Information for X-ray Imaging Device Premarket Notifications* outlines FDA's current thinking on information that should be provided in premarket notifications for x-ray imaging devices with indications for use in pediatric populations in efforts to reduce the amount of unnecessary radiation to pediatric patients through medical imaging. A planned draft guidance document is near completion that will express FDA's current thinking on extrapolation of adult efficacy data for approved devices, in order to extend claims to pediatric patients.

Two major initiatives from CDRH's Office of Science and Engineering Laboratories (OSEL) involve dosing devices and thermometers. Devices which deliver liquid formulations of varying degrees of viscosity can sometimes measure inaccurately and lead to incorrect dosing. OSEL is also working on improving the accuracy of thermometers that are less accurate in their "fast" modes.

2.4.2.2. Pediatric Device Consortia Grants Program
Linda Ulrich, M.D., Director, PDC Grant Program, OOPD, FDA

Background

PMDSIA enacted in 2007, called for an enhanced Federal response to pediatric device needs and required, among other things, the establishment of non-profit pediatric device consortia. The PDC consist of groups of organizations and individuals with diverse experience and skill sets that work together to apply resources and expertise towards the common goal of developing medical devices for children.

Technical Overview

Consortia are a critical tool for device development; they provide a place for innovators to obtain an upfront assessment of their proposed ideas. Each consortium brings together advising services in the areas of legal/ intellectual property, engineering, scientific, business, clinical, and regulatory expertise. Ideally, these groups consider and advise on business feasibility and regulatory planning at all phases of device development.

The major portion of Dr. Ulrich's presentation provided information about the PDC Grants Program which has awarded over $14 million in grants in its first five years since its inception via three cycles of grant competition. Under FDASIA, the PDC program was authorized to receive up to $5.25 million per year; however, the program currently receives funding of $3 million per year. This program does not invest in specific products, but rather focuses on funding consortia that support pediatric device developers. At the time of Dr. Ulrich's presentation the PDC Grants Program had assisted more than 260 proposed pediatric medical device projects, the majority of which were very early stage projects. Of the assisted projects, more than 110 currently remain active.

2.4.2.3. Medical Device Innovation Program

Michelle McMurry-Heath, M.D., Ph.D., Associate Director for Science, CDRH, FDA

Background

The Medical Device Innovation Consortium (MDIC) is a non-profit 501(c)(3)[36] organization that operates in partnership with FDA and others to improve the medical technology environment. It was launched in December 2011, and has 35 members which include the Centers for Medicare and Medicaid Services (CMS), NIH, FDA, NORD, the PEW Foundation, the Patient Centered Outcome Research Institute (PCORI), and private groups including companies such as Johnson & Johnson, Boston Scientific, Becton Dickinson, and St. Jude Medical.

Technical Overview

This presentation focused on ways in which members of the MDIC work together to try to reduce the time and resources needed for any single company or any single group of researchers to bring new solutions to patients, including those with PRD. The MDIC works on identifying key regulatory science (i.e., the tools, standards, and approaches needed to develop a new medical device, to test that the device is performing as predicted, and to regulate the device for safety and effectiveness) hurdles in device development, and members collaborate to address these hurdles with the hope of more research in this area being funded.

CDRH regulatory science priorities include improving the health of pediatric and other populations through a reduction in the time and cost of device development and review, thereby getting safer devices to market more quickly and efficiently. Developing the MDIC as a public-private partnership among industry, FDA, other agencies, and non-profits assures that no group alone must support the total product lifecycle (i.e., discovery and ideation to the approval and postmarket) of a given device. CDRH recognized a distinct need for public-private partnerships in the early "pre-competitive" space of technology innovation. The consortium has initially chosen to focus on three key areas, (1) improving computer models for device development, (2) clinical trial design and reform, and (3) patientcenteredness in medical device development.

2.4.2.4. Innovation Pathway

Murray Sheldon, M.D., Associate Director for Technology and Innovation, CDRH, FDA This session can be viewed in its entirety at Webcast Part 1.

Background

CDRH's Innovation Pathway was developed to help improve FDA's effort to advance medical device innovation in the U.S. market. It was noted that start-up investment in medical device innovation in the United States had decreased by more than 70% since its peak in 2007. Regulatory challenges (38%), reimbursement concerns (18%), and clinical trial issues (14%) were cited in a survey (NVCA MedIC Vital Signs Report, October 2011) as factors having the highest impact on companies' decisions to move biomedical investment (including medical devices) outside the United States. The Innovation Pathway was designed to help bring the United States back into the forefront of global device development.

Technical Overview

FDA acknowledges real or perceived problems in the current landscape of medical device development and is concerned that as more initial clinical testing of novel devices has moved to non-U.S. sites, device innovation may follow. This can lead to devices that are exclusively developed for non-U.S. markets. There is a growing concern regarding the time lag between available products in the United States and in other parts of the world. The Innovation Pathway was developed to address these issues through three goals.

The first is to shorten the time from concept to commercialization. This involves understanding the issues of preclinical testing, clinical trials, reimbursements, marketing, manufacturing, etc., and emphasizing that product developers contact FDA earlier, through pre-submission programs. The pathway also seeks to improve benefit-risk assessment, primarily based on the patients' perspective. The second goal is to transform the user experience through collaboration to form "one team" with FDA, in order to create a roadmap that will help sponsors understand the pathway for regulatory approval or clearance. The third goal is to make decisions that create forward momentum. If development comes to the point it can no longer move forward from a regulatory perspective, this must be communicated quickly and effectively, and with potential paths forward offered.

Examples of successes under these goals include the use of PMA supplements in lieu of original PMA applications for pediatric-sized heart valves. The End Stage Renal Disease Challenge, a pilot program for innovative devices that address end-stage renal disease and the Entrepreneurs in Residence Program, a time-limited recruitment of world-class entrepreneurs and innovators to join highly-qualified internal government employees in the development of solutions in areas that impact innovation.

2.4.3. Day 3, Session 3: HUD/ HDE Discussion

Moderator: Victoria Wagman, Health Scientist, Office of the Center Director, CDRH. This session can be viewed in its entirety at Webcast Part 2.

2.4.3.1. Humanitarian Use Devices

Eric Chen, M.S., Director, HUD Program, OOPD, FDA.

Background

A HUD is a device that is intended to benefit patients by treating or diagnosing a disease or condition that affects or is manifested in fewer than 4,000 individuals in the United States per year. To obtain approval for a HUD, an HDE application is submitted to FDA. An HDE is similar in both form and content to a PMA application, but is exempt from the effectiveness requirements of a PMA. The HDE process is described in greater detail in the summary of the next session.

Technical Overview

Eric Chen reviewed the HUD/HDE program, established to encourage the development of medical devices for rare diseases. To be eligible for an HDE, a sponsor must first request that the device be designated by OOPD as a HUD. In reviewing a HUD designation request, OOPD will evaluate the disease or condition, the scientific rationale and the population estimate (i.e., incidence) to determine if the device qualifies. In order to define the intended population for use, OOPD will focus on how the device works to treat or diagnose the disease or condition. If the sponsor proposes that only a subset of patients may use the device, then the sponsor must provide adequate information to demonstrate that the subset is considered an "orphan subset". The session also included a discussion of some of the issues associated with designations, for example, the distinction between designating therapeutic devices versus diagnostic devices.

Once a HUD designation has been obtained, an HDE application must be submitted to CDRH or CBER in order to get the HUD to market. Obtaining an HUD designation does not guarantee approval of the HDE application. From 1996 through November 2013, 318 HUD designation requests had been submitted; 207 of these devices received HUD designation, and 58 HDEs had been approved. Eight of these approved HDEs were authorized to make a profit.

2.4.3.2. Humanitarian Device Exemptions (HDE) Overview

Captain Nicole Wolanski, Captain, USPHS, Director, Premarket Approval Section, Office of Device Evaluation, CDRH, FDA.

Background

As mentioned in Presentation I of Session 3, an HDE authorizes the marketing of a HUD. An HDE exempts the effectiveness standard FDA generally requires prior to device approval, thereby helping to speed a potential new product to market.

Technical Overview

Captain Wolanski presented the process of submitting an application for HDE and reviewed the statutory changes allowing HUDs to earn a profit. In order to qualify for review as an HDE device, a sponsor must demonstrate that (1) the product is designated as a HUD device, (2) the device could not otherwise be brought to market through a 510(k) clearance or PMA and, (3) no comparable device is currently available. The session included a description of what an HDE submission should include; an HDE checklist for filing decision is available to aid in this process. HDE approval is based upon, (1) safety, i.e., that the device does not expose patients to unreasonable risk of illness or injury, and (2) a finding that the probable benefit of the device outweighs the risks of using the device, taking into account the probable risks and benefits of alternative therapies. After HDE approval, IRB approval is required prior to a device's use (except in emergency situations). Labeling for HDE approved devices must clearly identify a device as an HUD and state that effectiveness for the indication has not been demonstrated.

Currently, an HUD is eligible to be sold for profit if the device is intended for the treatment or diagnosis of a disease or condition that occurs in pediatric patients or in a pediatric subpopulation, and is labeled as such; **or** the device is intended for the treatment or diagnosis of a disease or condition that does not occur in pediatric patients or that occurs in pediatric patients in such numbers that the development of the device for such patients is impossible, highly impracticable, or unsafe.

2.4.3.3. IRB Oversight of Humanitarian Use Devices (What's an IRB to Do?)

Robert "Skip" Nelson, M.D., Ph.D., Deputy Director and Senior Pediatric Ethicist, OPT, FDA.

Background

FDA issued a guidance document to answer commonly asked questions about HUDs and HDE entitled, Guidance for HDE Holders, Institutional Review Boards (IRBs), Clinical Investigators, and Food and Drug Administration Staff – Humanitarian Device Exemption (HDE) Regulation: Questions and Answers. A HUD can be used in two general ways, as part of: (1) **medical practice**: A HUD can be used according to its approved labeling and indication(s) to treat or diagnose patients. It can also be used "off label" as part of medical practice; or (2) **clinical investigation**: A HUD can be used in a clinical investigation (i.e., collection of safety and effectiveness data). A HUD may be studied in a clinical investigation in accordance with its approved indication(s) or for a different indication.

Technical Overview

Dr. Nelson's presentation focused on regulations governing the role of IRBs with regard to HUD use.

When a HUD is to be used in medical practice, IRBs should follow the review criteria at 21 CFR 56.111 and elsewhere in Part 56 as much as possible. The IRB should review the risks to patients that are found in the product labeling, ensure the risks are minimized, and evaluate whether the risks are reasonable in relation to the proposed use of the device. Prior to HDE approval, any clinical investigation using the device must be conducted in accordance with the IDE regulations (21 CFR Part 812) and must have IRB approval. Following HDE approval, the HDE holder may collect safety and effectiveness data on the HUD, in a clinical investigation for the HDE-approved indication(s) without an IDE. Clinical investigation of a HUD for an indication different from the HDE-approved indication(s) must be conducted in compliance with IDE regulations, and IRB approval (21 CFR Part 56) and protection of human subjects (21 CFR Part 50) are required.

2.4.4. Day 3, Session 4: Engineering Considerations

Moderator: Eric Chen, M.S., Director, HUD Program, OOPD, FDA This session can be viewed in its entirety at Webcast Part 2

2.4.4.1. Engineering Considerations

Christy Foreman, M.S., Director, Office of Device Evaluation, CDRH, FDA

General Overview

The *Premarket Assessment of Pediatric Medical Devices* guidance document defines pediatric patients as ≤ 21 years of age at the time of diagnosis or treatment. Necessary factors in building an effective device suitable for a pediatric patient include more than simply building a smaller version of an adult device.

Technical Overview

Christy Foreman's presentation addressed engineering considerations specific to developing pediatric devices. A typical pediatric modification to an adult device, besides a reduction in size, might include attenuation of electrical output. Stresses on a device as a child grows or that result from a child's activity level need to be kept in mind. Engineers must also consider the impact a device can have on a child's development. Because of difficulties in conducting clinical trials, most questions are answered via bench testing. Computational modeling of medical devices can decrease the amount of bench testing needed. FDA is interested working with sponsors who are developing pediatric medical devices to discuss such considerations early in the development process. The general principles of device review that exists for all medical devices also apply for pediatric medical devices.

2.4.5. Day 3, Session 5: Clinical Trials Issues Panel

Moderator: Markham Luke, M.D., Ph.D., Deputy Director, Office of Device Evaluation, CDRH, FDA This session can be viewed in its entirety at Webcast Part 3.

2.4.5.1. Trial Design Considerations

John Laschinger, M.D., Medical Officer, Structural Heart Devices Branch, CDRH.

Background

A **significant risk (Class III) device** presents a potential for serious risk to the health, safety, or welfare of a subject. Examples include sutures, cardiac pacemakers, hydrocephalus shunts, and orthopedic implants. Advice on distinguishing between significant risk and non-significant risks studies are outlined in the guidance document titled, *Significant Risk and Nonsignificant Risk Medical Device Studies*.

Technical Overview

Dr. Laschinger's presentation focused on clinical trial design considerations for significant risk devices.

The approval process for a significant risk device is divided into two phases, the pre-clinical phase and the clinical phase. The pre-clinical phase is designed to show that the device is safe through a combination of bench tests, animal studies, computational modeling, biocompatibility, toxicity, sterilization, and manufacturing. The pivotal clinical trial is to obtain valid scientific evidence, and generally includes three phases: the design, conduct, and analysis of the trial. The process can be facilitated through early communication with FDA.

Dr. Laschinger discussed an evidence hierarchy, with order of desirability from most to least that includes: prospective randomized controlled studies; partially controlled studies; studies without matched controls; prospective registry studies; meta-analyses of large case series; physiologic study; retrospective case series; and expert opinion. He noted that pediatric device and HDE trials generally are not subjected to prospective randomized trials because the patient numbers are too small.

A strong trial shows a device's benefits outweigh the risks. Benefits should be represented as clinically meaningful in terms of type, magnitude, and probability, and the data cited for these claims should be reproducible, generalizable, and durable. Patient factors include tolerance to disease, symptoms, disease severity/chronicity, and available drug options. Risk considerations include harmful events, their type, number, severity, probability, duration, and mitigation.

2.4.5.2. Extrapolation Issues: Bayesian Methods for Making Inferences About Rare Diseases in Pediatric Populations

Laura Thompson, Ph.D., Division of Biostatistics, CDRH, FDA.

Background

Bayesian methods combine prior information, such as that gathered in previous trials on a related product or the same product on a different population, with current trial data on an endpoint of interest (e.g., an adverse event rate), in order to form conclusions about the endpoint.

Technical Overview

Bayesian statistical methods can be used to make inferences about rare diseases in pediatric populations. Challenging issues with studying rare diseases in pediatric populations include dealing with small sample sizes and estimation of the occurrence of rare events. Bayesian methods can be used to overcome these issues. They provide a way to learn from evidence as it accumulates. A final guidance document on Bayesian statistics titled, *Guidance for the Use of Bayesian Statistics in Medical Device Clinical Trials* is available.

Bayesian methods can be used to gain statistical power by combining data from prior and current trials (i.e., borrowing strength) when dealing with the challenge of small sample sizes. The extent of borrowing from prior data depends on the similarity between the prior and current trials (i.e., exchangeability between trials). To the extent that prior and current trial results differ, borrowing strength weakens the process. In the case of borrowing (i.e., extrapolating) prior adult data to be combined with current pediatric trial data, the forthcoming draft guidance document, *Extrapolation of Data for Pediatric Uses of Medical Devices*, introduces a framework for decisions about whether borrowing or extrapolating from adult data is appropriate.

Adaptive or flexible designs are discussed in FDA's recently released guidance document, *Design Considerations for Pivotal Clinical Investigations for Medical Devices*. These are trial designs that allow a prospectively planned opportunity for modification during the course of a trial, for instance a change of entry criteria, dropping/adding an arm, change randomization ratio, sample size re-estimation, and early stops for effectiveness or futility. These designs are available for pediatric studies and can be useful in, among other purposes, the performance of an adequate trial with fewer patients.

2.4.5.3. Patient Registries as a Prelude to Clinical Trials and Post-Approval Studies

Stephen Groft, PharmD, Director, Office of Rare Diseases Research, National Center for Advancing Translational Sciences (NCATS), NIH.

Background
A **patient registry** is a list or database of patient information that scientists and researchers can use to keep track of patients who have participated in clinical trials, including all relevant study information, to monitor potential long-term health effects of a given therapy and shape future clinical trials.

Technical Overview
Dr. Groft's presentation focused on the value of patient registries in moving clinical research forward.

Patient registries can: (1) improve patient recruitment; (2) identify possible patient cohorts for study; (3) serve as a lead-in to natural history studies; (4) integrate patient reported and clinical data from multiple sources into a single repository; (5) stimulate new research and lead to new scientific insights; and (6) enhance creative data mining within and across disorders. When developing a new registry, the following should be taken into consideration: (1) the purpose of the registry; (2) the process of data (identified and de-identified) collection, management, and analyses across multiple platforms; (3) the data curator's role, (4) the type of informed consent needed (restricted or broad access); (5) IRB and Federal Information Security Management Act requirements; (6) data sources (patient, family, caregiver, and healthcare provider); (7) uses of common and unique data elements; and (8) options for data updates. It is important to further develop partnerships and collaborations between stakeholders in the rare disease community, and to agree upon the use of common and unique data elements in order to contribute to the sharing of data.

2.4.6. Day 3, Session 6: Needs Assessment
Moderators: Debra Lewis, OD, MBA, Deputy Director, OOPD, FDA and Eric Chen, M.S., Director, HUD Program, OOPD, FDA
This session can be viewed in its entirety at Webcast Part 3.

2.4.6.1. Medical Devices for Rare Diseases: FDA/NIH Needs Assessment Project
Gayatri R. Rao, M.D., J.D., Director, OOPD, FDA

Background
An Institute of Medicine (IOM) Rare Diseases and Orphan Products Report (2010) recommended that "FDA and NIH should collaborate on an assessment of unmet device needs and priorities relevant to rare diseases. That assessment should focus on the most plausible areas of unmet need, identify impediments

to meeting these needs, and examine options for overcoming impediments and stimulating high priority innovations."

Technical Overview

Dr. Rao discussed FDA's plans to conduct a medical device needs assessment for rare disease patients in order to document the compelling need for devices in this patient population. Its primary focus is on identifying device needs for rare diseases, rather than barriers to development. Multiple stakeholders for the project include the rare disease and pediatric patient groups, industry, clinicians, and professional organizations. While the IOM recommendation was not specific to PRD, FDA's needs assessment will have a sub-focus on the pediatric population. The scope of the initiative will span across a broad spectrum of medical disciplines, rather than providing an in-depth concentration on a single discipline (e.g., only cardiovascular device needs). Different approaches to conducting the needs assessment were discussed, including surveys, conducting targeted focus group interviews, and public meetings. The needs assessment experiences from the audience were shared.

2.4.7. Day 3, Session 7: Diagnostic Devices

Moderator: Markham Luke, M.D., Ph.D., Deputy Director, Office of Device Evaluation, CDRH, FDA This session can be viewed in its entirety at: Webcast Part 4

2.4.7.1. Considerations for Diagnostics

Alberto Gutierrez, Ph.D., Director, Office of In Vitro Diagnostics and Radiological Health, CDRH, FDA.

Background

Diagnostic devices play an important role in the correct identification of a disease and in helping to determine treatment. FDA estimates that more than 70% of all medical decisions require some type of diagnostic test, so these devices comprise a large portion of our medical care system.

Technical Overview

Dr. Gutierrez explained that risk is determined differently for diagnostics than for therapeutic devices.

In determining the risk of a diagnostic device, FDA considers the risk of an erroneous result, be it a false positive or a false negative. Thus, the safety and the efficacy of the device are intricately linked. It is very difficult to determine safety, without determining some kind of efficacy. This makes applying the HDE approval process particularly difficult for diagnostic devices because efficacy is not a determining factor for approval in the HDE pathway. For this reason, it is generally easier to evaluate diagnostic devices through the 510(k) process or through a down-classification to a Class II device.

2.4.8. Day 3, Session 8: What Could be Done? Incentives and Otherwise

Moderator: Jacqueline Ryan, M.D., Medical Officer, Division of Anesthesia, General Hospital, Infection Control and Dental Devices, CDRH, FDA.

This session can be viewed in its entirety at: Webcast Part 4.

2.4.8.1. Stakeholder Perspectives

In this session representatives from various stakeholder groups provided their perspectives on what could be done to help advance the development of devices for PRD.

Tamar Magarik Haro, Assistant Director, Department of Federal Affairs, American Academy of Pediatrics noted that earlier in the meeting it was stated that the PDC Grant Program is only receiving $3 million of its authorized maximum $5.25 million in Federal appropriations. She noted the PDC is a "small but mighty" program and that it is imperative for it to be fully funded. She also noted that payer and insurance issues continue to plague advancement of devices. Continued denials of payment from insurance companies on approved HUD devices and a lack of understanding by payers about HDEs are true impediments. Ms. Haro voiced a need for the upcoming extrapolation guidance that was discussed earlier in the meeting. Ms. Haro stated that the statutory mandate for IRB review of approved HDE devices should be reconsidered. Also, Ms. Haro noted a need to overcome challenges to FDA's ability to find and maintain pediatric expertise on its advisory committees.

Michael C. Morton, V.P. Regulatory Affairs of Medtronic, Inc. For AdvaMed - Advanced Medical Technology Association noted a need for flexible regulatory models, so that FDA is authorized to use valid scientific evidence other than well-controlled trials. While acknowledging a great deal has been accomplished by FDA in the area of pediatric devices for rare diseases, he also noted a need for further HDE/HUD program clarifications, for example, how "probable benefit" is defined. He also suggested FDA use of an ombudsman program, dedicated to orphan rare diseases and pediatrics. He also recommended greater use of early stage meetings between sponsors and FDA when sponsors are developing a product. Referring to Dr. Geiger's presentation which demonstrated a variety of devices that are too big for children being used anyway because that is all surgeons have, Mr. Morton also raised the idea of creating more clarity around rules regarding custom devices.

Diane Dorman, Vice President for Public Policy NORD said she believes it is critically important to ensure that the incentives contained in the Orphan Drug Act remain strong, in order to continue to encourage development of products and to increase research for rare diseases. Commenting on the presentation in this meeting by FDA's Gayatri Rao, Ms. Dorman noted that a comprehensive needs assessment for devices for rare diseases is an important priority. She also noted the confusion associated with the requirement for IRB review of approved HUDs and the potential hurdle it creates for reimbursement. Ms. Dorman echoed earlier advice with regard to FDA engaging sponsors early in the product development process, but added that this early engagement should be extended to include the patient community as well.

Steve Hirschfeld, MD, PhD, CAPT, USPHS, Associate Director for Clinical Research, NICHD, NIH said that in every government funding agency, particularly NIH, there are funds set aside for small businesses to conduct innovation research and technology transfer. For this reason, he suggested the establishment of public-private partnerships to provide funding. He concurred with the need for a comprehensive rare disease needs assessment but acknowledged the complexities involved with conducting one. Dr. Hirschfeld also recommended the need to think globally because while the market size in the United States may be small, in other parts of the world there may be patient populations that raise the market size for any effective intervention.

2.4.9. Summary of Comments from the Lunchtime Breakout Sessions

During the lunchtime breakout sessions, participants discussed specialty-specific issues related to medical devices for treatment of PRD. The participants were asked to provide examples of existing medical devices that have the best potential for modification to address the need for treatment or diagnosis of a disease in the PRD population and to state if no device is currently available to address this need.

The orthopedic group provided the example of growth modulation as an important area for further modification. The general surgery participants provided multiple examples, which included drug delivery pumps, intrathecal devices, electrosurgical devices, devices used in minimally invasive surgery, and surgical staplers. The gastrointestinal and renal discussants suggested that pH probes and reflux devices could potentially be modified and the cardiology participants provided the examples of stents, valves, defibrillators, and catheters. The neurology and physical medicine rehabilitation participants provided the example of neurostimulation devices.

When asked what are the best ways to foster networking across agencies, academia, professional societies, and patient groups to address the medical device needs of pediatric patients with rare diseases, most of the participants in all groups suggested that outreach by FDA to individual professional societies and other stakeholders would be best. The groups also listed outreach to consortia as an important focus.

2.4.10. Summary of Comments from the Public Dockets for Day 3

Two comments were submitted to the public docket. Again, the majority of the comments echoed the discussion and suggestions expressed by panelists and other participants during the meetings.

Additional suggestions include: the creation of a tax credit for HUDs that is similar to the tax credits that exist for orphan drugs; the creation of an orphan/pediatric ombudsman in CDRH; the ability to extrapolate clinical data between different sizes of the same device based on engineering testing and other nonclinical data; and the creation of a compassionate use orphan/pediatric device provision to be applied in certain HUD/HDE pathway situations (i.e., the number of patients affected annually are too few to justify the expense).

Also, one comment suggested a future FDA guidance document to address the evidence needed to meet the probable benefit standard for HDE.

3. STRATEGIC PLAN: ACCELERATING THE DEVELOPMENT OF THERAPIES FOR PRD

The Strategic Plan sets out FDA's plan for accelerating therapies for PRD. The Strategic Plan is intended to assist FDA and the PRD community to focus together on the most efficient path to the stated goal.

3.1. Workgroups Formed to Develop Strategic Plan

Multiple FDA workgroups contributed to development of the Workshops[37] and formulating this Strategic Plan. The drugs/biologics Strategic Plan

Workgroup was comprised of FDA representatives from OOPD, OPT, CBER, CDER (including representatives from the Rare Disease Program [RDP], the Pediatric and Maternal Health Staff [PMHS], the Office of Hematology and Oncology Products [OHOP], and the Office of Communications [OCOMM]). The Devices Strategic Plan Workgroup was comprised of FDA representatives from OOPD, OPT, CBER, CDRH, and CDER OCOMM. OOPD took the lead in coordinating this strategic plan. The Office of Policy (OP) was consulted for guidance in its structure and approach.

3.2. Strategic Plan: Primary Goal and Four Objectives

The Strategic Plan Workgroups began with the stated goal of identifying strategies "to encourage and accelerate the development of new therapies (drugs, biologics, and devices) for PRD", mirroring the FDASIA requirement.

Using the input from the workshops and the workgroup members' knowledge of pediatrics and rare diseases, four objectives were formulated which categorize the overarching elements of the product development process.

The four objectives follow:

1. Enhance foundational and translational science for PRD;
2. Strengthen communication, collaboration, and partnering for PRD within and outside FDA;
3. Advance the use of regulatory science to aid clinical trial design and performance for PRD; and
4. Enhance FDA's review process for PRD products.

Individual strategies to advance development of therapies for PRD were grouped under each objective.

The four objectives are in the same order as the product development process. The workgroups recognize that the boundaries between the objectives are not completely distinct and that there may be overlap amongst them. Similarly, some of the strategies have the potential to be placed under more than one objective. This is seen as a positive, in that the strategies can positively affect more than one area of the development process. Each strategy was grouped under the objective that the workgroup members believed will be most affected.

Further, the strategies strengthen and enhance the initiatives FDA is undertaking that address the stated goal and objectives. The strategies range from those specifically targeted to therapies for PRD to those of a broader scope which do not have a specific pediatric deliverable, but have the ability to support the development of new therapies for PRD. The strategies are separated into drug/biologic and device categories.

The FDA review process of the fourth objective signifies the point in time when an application for marketing approval is submitted to FDA. The earlier FDA review processes, e.g., investigational device exemption [IDE] and IND, are integrated into the first three objectives. These objectives are in alignment with many of FDA's draft Core Mission Objectives. A list of FDA's draft Core Mission Goals and Objectives can be found in Appendix 1and a crosswalk demonstrating the linkage between this Strategic Plan's objectives and the relevant FDA draft Core Mission Objectives can be found in Appendix 2.

Table 1 lists the goal, objectives and strategies of this strategic plan.

Table 1. Goal, Objectives, and Strategies

GOAL	
To encourage and accelerate the development of new therapies for PRD	
Objective 1: Enhance foundational and translational science for PRD	
Drugs/Biologics	**Strategies**
	• Facilitate the conduct of natural history studies for PRD • Publish draft guidance on common issues in rare disease drug development
Devices	• Identify unmet PRD needs in medical device development • Refine and expand the use of computational modeling • Explore the use of registry data for use in both premarket and postmarket evaluation of medical devices intended for pediatric populations
Objective 2: Strengthen communication, collaboration and partnering for PRD within and outside FDA	
Drugs/Biologics and Devices	**Strategies**
	• Continue to foster interagency (public-public) and public-private partnerships • Continue to foster international collaborations • Continue to foster Intra-Agency collaborations

GOAL		
To encourage and accelerate the development of new therapies for treating pediatric rare diseases		
Objective 3: Advance the use of regulatory science to aid clinical trial design and performance for PRD		
Drugs/Biologics	**Strategies**	
	• Develop additional FDA guidance relevant to PRD • Increase engagement of the Study Endpoints and Labeling Development (SEALD) Staff early in instrument development to navigate COA process	
	• Facilitate increasing the knowledge of biamarkers and COAs useful for PRD, including engaging with investigators and organizations in biomarker and clinical outcome qualification programs to advise during their development • Develop training programs for pediatric clinical investigators • Explore modeling and simulation approaches (e.g., physiologically-based pharnnacokinetic [PBPK] models) to provide preliminary data for drugs used in PRD to inform the design and conduct of PK/PD studies and other clinical trials for investigational drugs in PRD populations	
Devices	• Develop expedited approval pathway for certain devices intended to treat unmet medical needs • Evaluate the results of an analysis of approved medical devices to explore the feasibility of shifting some premarket data requirements to the postmarket setting for future medical devices • Support the development of Medical Device Development Tools to improve clinical trial performance • Develop curriculum for undergraduate/graduate studies to increase understanding of regulatory approval process for device development	
General	• Use FDA web-based resources to update and expand awareness of for PRD product development issues • Increase awareness in pediatric rare disease researchers, product developers, and patient community of funding opportunities through OPD grant program	

(Continued)

Objective 4: Enhance FDA's review process for PRD products	
Drugs/Biologics	**Strategies**
	• Foster FDA's efforts to obtain patients' and caregivers' perspectives for incorporation in drug development • Further develop and implement a structured approach to benefit-risk assessment in the drug review process • issue Rare Pediatric Disease PRV draft guidance document
	• Continue reviewer training for rare and PRD • Explore potential for innovation in data analysis
Devices	• Further develop methods to implement the incorporation of patient preferences into assessments of premarket approval and de novo classifications of devices • Establish a patient engagement panel as part of CDRH's Medical Advisory Committee • Analyze the HDE process for medical devices that diagnosis and treat PRD • Set standards for whole genorne sequencing that can be used as a comparator
General	• Continue to enhance FDA's expertise to review innovative products

3.3. Objective 1: Enhance Foundational and Translational Science for PRD

3.3.1. Drugs/Biologics

3.3.1.1. Strategy: Facilitate the Conduct of Natural History Studies for PRD

Understanding the natural history of a disease serves as a foundation for the development of medical products to treat it and contributes to all phases of development. For example, a well characterized natural history can help identify biomarkers and drug targets, as well as guide clinical trial design and the selection of clinically meaningful endpoints.

Children affected by rare diseases are usually a small, heterogeneous population. Many rare diseases that affect children lack a comprehensive characterization of their natural history. More natural history studies conducted for PRD would increase the natural history knowledge base and serve to advance the development of drugs to treat them.

There are various types of natural history studies (e.g., retrospective, prospective, cross-sectional, and prospective longitudinal), each with their strengths and weaknesses. When conducting a natural history study, the data elements which will best serve the disease being studied, the collection and storage of the data, as well as the ethics of its conduct, must be taken into consideration. Therefore, FDA encourages sponsors to engage the agency in discussions regarding the design and conduct of natural history studies, as these studies can have a broad applicability to different modes of treatment. FDA recognizes the need to provide a clear avenue for this communication to occur since these discussions may not be related to a specific drug, and, therefore, do not fit into the existing framework for regulatory submissions.

The Critical Path Innovation Meeting (CPIM) is one such forum for these high-level discussions to occur. The CPIM is a recently-launched FDA program that gives investigators from industry, academia, government, and patient advocacy groups the opportunity to meet with FDA to discuss proposals for innovative tools and methods in drug development, which includes natural history study design and implementation. For example, the Agency met with an external stakeholder to discuss natural history studies for adrenoleukodystrophy, a rare X-linked disorder that generally causes rapid degeneration to a vegetative state in childhood.

Other examples of potential topics for discussion at the CPIM include potential biomarkers and COAs in the early phase of development and not ready for their qualification programs, emerging technologies or new uses of existing technologies, and innovative conceptual approaches to clinical trial design and analysis.

The discussions at a CPIM are nonbinding and do not substitute for other types of meetings (e.g., preIND, IND, pre-Biologic License Application, etc.). Requests for the meeting are received by CDER's Office of Translational Sciences (OTS) and expertise from CDER and other centers is provided. Increasing the awareness of CPIM and the opportunities it provides should facilitate the design and conduct of more natural history studies capable of informing drug development for PRD. FDA plans to issue a draft guidance document regarding the CPIM to help increase awareness and facilitate the usefulness of this resource.

3.3.1.2. Strategy: Publish Draft Guidance on Common Issues in Rare Disease Drug Development

Common issues in drug development for rare diseases include the small numbers of patients with the individual disease available for study, phenotypic heterogeneity, and often, a lack of regulatory precedence. The lack of regulatory precedence often means there is a lack of accepted endpoints, outcome assessment measures, instruments, and tools for the study of the disease.

FDA plans to issue guidance to facilitate understanding of these common rare disease issues. Although there is no deliverable specific to pediatrics associated with this document, some of the common issues in rare disease drug development, such as the small numbers of patients available for study, are compounded when developing drugs for children. Therefore, FDA advice on managing these common issues should be helpful to developers of therapies for PRD.

3.3.2. Devices

3.3.2.1. Strategy: Identify Unmet PRD Needs in Medical Device Development

The identification of unmet PRD needs in medical device development will put FDA in a position to better coordinate efforts of stakeholders, device manufacturers, and FDA staff to promote new device development and proper labeling of existing medical devices for pediatric use.

FDA (OOPD and CDRH), along with NIH, plans to conduct a medical device needs assessment for rare disease patients in order to document the compelling need for devices in this patient population. FDA's needs assessment will have a sub-focus on the pediatric population. Multiple stakeholders for the project include the rare disease and pediatric patient groups, industry, clinicians, and professional organizations.

In addition, in January 2014, FDA issued a Final Rule[38] regarding pediatric uses of medical devices that require persons who submit certain medical device applications to include, if readily available, a description of any pediatric subpopulations that suffer from the disease or condition that the device is intended to treat, diagnose or cure, and the number of affected pediatric patients. Although the pediatric uses information is not specific to rare diseases, the unmet needs in medical device development for PRD will be captured, and implementation of this Final Rule will help further the development of medical devices for them. A final guidance document, *Providing Information about*

Pediatric Uses of Medical Devices, describes how to compile and submit the required, readily available pediatric use information.

3.3.2.2. *Strategy*: *Refine* **and Expand the Use of Computational Modeling**

FDA plans to further refine and expand its use of computational modeling. Computational modeling uses computer-based, mathematical techniques and can predict how a device will perform before a single prototype is produced. These techniques can be used to anticipate the performance of medical devices when they're used in various patient groups, including children. For example, computational modeling is being used to predict the best ways to defibrillate children, who are poorly served by existing defibrillation devices, which have only been optimized and studied for use in adults.

Computational models can speed the design and testing of new and improved devices by allowing developers to test their ideas on the screen. Testing devices via computational modeling also enables the specialization of devices when the disease prevalence does not permit widespread clinical trials, such as in PRD. Further, the risk to patients in clinical trials can be reduced by first testing designs in the virtual human. These attributes of computational modeling have the potential to give rise to new companies and allow existing companies to work more efficiently, expediently, and safely, which should stimulate further development of medical devices for PRD.

3.3.2.3. Strategy: Explore the Use of Registry Data for Use in Both Premarket and Postmarket Evaluation of Medical Devices Intended for Pediatric Populations

CDRH is exploring the idea of using registry data to facilitate market access for innovative products, e.g., serve as the comparison group of "control arm" in scientific studies evaluating device performance. CDRH is also exploring appropriate use of registry data to assist in studies for new uses of existing devices and to possibly expand labeled indications to new patient populations. These efforts may be particularly helpful to the assessments of benefit-risk in small populations, such as children with rare diseases.

3.4. Objective 2: Strengthen Communication, Collaboration and Partnering for PRD within and outside FDA

3.4.1. Drugs/Biologics and Devices

3.4.1.1. Strategy: Continue to Foster Interagency (Public-Public) and Public-Private Partnerships

FDA maintains many partnerships and collaborations with other governmental agencies and private organizations which help to stimulate the development of products for rare diseases, including PRD. These relationships, which can leverage existing resources and incentives, are crucial to the success of developing products for PRD because most single entities (e.g., pharmaceutical manufacturer, academic institution, or governmental agency) may not have sufficient resources or expertise to independently develop products to treat PRD efficiently.

In addition, FDA participates with stakeholders in a number of workshops, meetings, and conferences to further educate and discuss challenges in the area of product development for rare diseases. FDA's presence can bring a needed perspective to allow for productive conversations on regulatory issues. Strengthening these partnerships and collaborations will further enable the development process for products for PRD through an exchange of advice and an increase in transparency, which can help to build a knowledge base for the generation of new programs.

Examples of FDA's partnerships and collaborations are listed below:

CDER's RDP and OTS are working with NORD and NIH's NCATS to develop natural history studies, including exploration of natural history study elements, designs and plans.

CBER is collaborating with NIH and the Health Resources and Services Administration on the Hematopoietic Stem Cell Transplantation Interagency Working Group. This working group reviews matters associated with hematopoietic stem cell transplantation to further their knowledge and use. CBER is also collaborating with NIH on a second working group, the CBER-FDA/National Institute of Neurological Disorder and Stroke-NIH Memorandum of Understanding Working Group which works to nurture expeditious translation of promising cellular/gene therapies to treat neurological diseases.

NCATS and OOPD are collaborating on "Discovering New Therapeutic Uses for Existing Molecules", which develops partnerships between pharmaceutical companies and the biomedical research community for therapy development. This repurposing initiative has the potential to save developer resources by using previous work as a head start on new PRD therapies.

CDER OHOP and CBER's OCTGT collaborates with oncology clinical trials networks (e.g., Children's Oncology Group and Pediatric Brain Tumor Consortium) on the identification of potentially relevant investigational products for early evaluation in the pediatric population and on design and conduct of "master" protocols, wherein multiple investigational drugs are studied across the same disease, or multiple agents directed at the same target are studied across multiple disease types.

PMHS and OPT collaborate with the Biotechnology Industry Organization and the Pharmaceutical Research and Manufacturers of America to discuss pediatric drug development, including rare diseases. Additional meetings are also planned to discuss important general pediatric drug development topics. These industry collaborations have been fostered in order to improve dialogue and facilitate early plans for collaborative interactions between academic investigators, clinical research networks, and international regulatory agencies when necessary.

Every month PMHS and OPT conduct a review with NICHD to assess progress made in the development of the identified "priority products (drugs)" list maintained by NICHD under BPCA. This program, known as the NIH/BPCA program, is intended to obtain pediatric data information that is adequate to support pediatric labeling for products in which there is little or no incentive for pharmaceutical manufacturers to do so (e.g., products with expired patents). Some of the products on the priority list are intended to treat PRD, which include important subpopulations such as neonates. Under this program, OPT, PMHS, and NICHD also meet with the academic subspecialty physicians to establish the priority list of products for study for their subspecialty. Data from studies of PRD may be incorporated into labeling following submission of these data by NIH to FDA under a newly-developed process.

There are many arenas in which FDA collaborates with external groups. For example, in an effort to identify trial issues contributing to the high failure rate for some pediatric trials, OPT established an Intergovernmental Personnel Act Mobility Program (IPA) Scholars program in 2005 with Duke University that allows academic physicians to assist in analysis of submitted pediatric trials. OPT has also established a consortium of six pediatric hospitals that work with FDA in identifying better ways to report safety issues that occur postmarketing. CDER, in collaboration with OPT, held the first Advancing the Development of Pediatric Therapeutics (ADEPT) Workshop in June, 2014 on Pediatric Bone Health. These workshops include regulatory, academic, industry and patient stakeholders and are intended to discuss important issues related to pediatric product development. More ADEPT workshops are scheduled for the future. Finally, OPT and PMHS have developed a monthly American Academy of Pediatrics Newsletter Column that directly communicates with practitioners to enhance their knowledge about changes in pediatric product development and the issues surrounding the studies required. Although these activities are not limited to PRD, these efforts are intended to advance overall pediatric product development which often includes discussions of PRD.

CDRH is working in partnership with the MDIC, an organization that includes other governmental agencies and private organizations that works to improve the medical technology environment. The MDIC works on identifying key regulatory science[39] hurdles in device development. Members address these hurdles with the hope that more research in this area will be funded.

The PDC Grants Program is administered by OOPD. The PDC brings together groups of device development experts with diverse experience and skill sets that apply their resources and expertise towards the common goal of developing medical devices for children.

Looking forward, there is a public health need as outlined by Congress and the IOM to study drugs in neonates. Research in the area of development of new technologies for newborn screening is advancing and most targeted conditions are rare diseases.[40] Therefore, more rare diseases may be diagnosed in the neonatal period. FDA is working with a number of external stakeholders to support a consortium model to advance the development of therapeutics for the neonatal population. There is recognition that this will require creative solutions engaging various drug development tools and methodologies, requiring input of a number of stakeholders across government, academia, industry, and professional societies.

3.4.1.2. Strategy: Continue to Foster International Collaborations

The pharmaceutical market has become more globalized and FDA maintains international collaborations which enable the exchange of information on development, safety, and effectiveness. Continuing to foster these collaborations should lead to increased global participation, along with a greater exchange of information, thereby advancing the development of these therapeutics. With regard to PRD, two monthly teleconferences are held between FDA and the EMA. One is in the area of pediatrics, initiated by OPT, and the other is in the area of orphan (i.e., rare disease) products, initiated by OOPD. These two areas are among others (e.g., genetic metabolic disorders, oncology, blood products, and biosimilars), identified as 'clusters' for regular exchanges to take place. OOPD's teleconferences with EMA may include difficult designation applications, divergent opinions, and rare disease initiatives and can result in joint rare disease projects, streamlining processes, and alignment of orphan designation issues.

The monthly teleconference initiated by OPT includes EMA, Japan (PMDA), Australia, and Canada's regulatory agencies. This teleconference allows for discussions on difficult applications, divergent opinions, and the details of Pediatric Investigational Plans (EMA) and Pediatric Study Plans (FDA). These shared perspectives and information can result in alignment, as far as possible, and expedite pediatric development plans. For example, in 2014 CDER and OPT worked with EMA to publish two documents on collaborative strategic approaches for development of rare diseases such as Gaucher's disease (issued by the EMA) and more common but difficult to enroll populations such as children with Type 2 Diabetes (accepted for publication by *Diabetes Care*). Also in 2014, CDER and OPT worked with EMA to complete a shared commentary document (shared with the sponsor) for the general approach to study products for the treatment of pediatric multiple sclerosis.

Furthermore, in 2014, OPT and CDER, in collaboration with EMA, Health Canada, and PMDA, published two manuscripts[41,42] on steps towards global harmonization for clinical development of medicines in pediatric ulcerative colitis. These manuscripts discussed the potential approaches to tackle the issues of study endpoints, biomarkers, data extrapolation, trial design, and pharmacokinetics in drug development.

Another international collaboration is FDA's collaboration with the International Rare Diseases Research Consortium (IRDiRC). The IRDiRC brings together researchers, regulatory agencies, advocacy groups and funding organizations investing in rare diseases. Some of the efforts undertaken through these collaborations are to explore gaps in the foundational science knowledge base of rare diseases (e.g., molecular and clinical characterization), research (i.e., preclinical, clinical and translational), and collaborative registries and biobanking efforts. Although not limited to PRD, IRDiRC efforts are intended to broadly contribute to rare disease research and product development, including those for PRD.

3.4.1.3. Strategy: Continue to foster Intra-Agency collaborations

To coordinate rare disease issues across the agency, the Rare Disease Council was established with representatives from different Offices and Centers including OOPD, CDER, CBER, CDRH, Center for Food Safety and Applied Nutrition (CFSAN), Office of Health and Constituent Affairs (OHCA), and

Office of Legislation. A representative from OPT will be added to the Council to facilitate pediatric perspectives. Continuing these efforts and addressing specific issues in PRD will help to advance therapies for these patients.

Further, CBER established a Rare Diseases Coordinating Committee within the Center to further facilitate and support the research, development, regulation, and approval of biological products and devices for the treatment of rare diseases, including pediatrics.

Additionally, the Agency will continue to support the work of the Pediatric Review Committee –PeRC, a cross-center committee that is responsible for the review of all pediatric product development, including PRD product development, under BPCA and PREA. The PeRC includes membership from CBER, CDER, Office of Chief Counsel, and OPT.

3.5. Objective 3: Advance the Use of Regulatory Science for PRD to Aid Clinical Trial Design and Performance

3.5.1. Drugs/Biologics

3.5.1.1. Strategy: Develop Additional FDA Guidance Relevant to PRD

In addition to guidance documents mentioned elsewhere in the Strategic Plan, several other draft guidance documents relevant to PRD are being developed.

FDA plans to publish two companion pediatric guidance documents to assist industry with pediatric product development under PREA and BPCA. The first guidance document is intended to assist industry in obtaining the data and information necessary to support use of drugs in pediatric populations by discussing selected clinical, scientific, and ethical issues. The second guidance document is focused on regulatory considerations and is intended to assist industry to comply with PREA and BPCA. Although orphan products (which include many products for PRD) are exempt from PREA, the availability of additional market exclusivity for PRD products under BPCA is an important incentive.

Another draft guidance document, *Pediatric Oncology Product Development*, is planned. Mechanisms of action for new drugs developed primarily for adult cancers may also predict potential relevance in certain pediatric cancers. Taking full advantage of pediatric legislative initiatives such as BPCA can incentivize and facilitate the early clinical evaluation of these drugs, which is especially pertinent to new molecularly targeted agents.

Expanded utilization of the Continuous Re-assessment Method (CRM) in pediatric phase 1 studies, especially when adequate toxicity and adult safety data exist, is encouraged to support dose finding efforts to permit earlier efficacy evaluation and to ultimately expedite the development of promising new drugs in the pediatric population.

The draft guidance document titled *Considerations for the Design of Early-Phase Clinical Trials of Cellular and Gene Therapy Products* was issued July 2013. The draft guidance includes a separate section on pediatrics. Cell and gene therapy products can be used to treat children with rare genetic diseases and FDA advice on the design of early-phase clinical trials to study the safety and effectiveness of these products will facilitate the development of these therapies. The Agency anticipates issuance of the final guidance document within two years.

Also issued in July 2013 was the draft guidance document titled *Pediatric Study Plans: Content of and Process for Submitting Initial Pediatric Study Plans and Amended Pediatric Study Plans*. This draft guidance document is intended to assist sponsors in the submission of an initial pediatric study plan (PSP) required under PREA and any amendments to the PSP by addressing who, when and what should be included in an initial PSP, as well as what should be included when requesting an amendment to the PSP.

3.5.1.2. Strategy: Increase Engagement of the Study Endpoints and Labeling Development (SEALD) Staff Early in Instrument Development to Navigate COA Process

The Study Endpoints team within CDER SEALD Staff ("Team") works to ensure that COAs are used appropriately in clinical trials to measure effectiveness endpoints and treatment benefit. Among other endeavors, the Team provides consultation and advice to FDA review staff on COA development, validation, and interpretation as effectiveness endpoints for use in clinical trials during product development. This refers to the development of COA instruments for a specific development program. The Team also manages and leads the COA Qualification Program (see Drug Development Tools Qualification Program), in which COAs can be developed for use across multiple development programs.

Promoting engagement with the Team early in the development process (prior to initiation of clinical trials if possible) will facilitate the process by allowing the Team to assist in the selection (or development) of appropriate clinical outcome assessments (i.e., patient, clinician, and observer reported outcome assessments, as well as performance measures). Their advice is intended to assist instrument developers in having the best chance at developing or selecting an instrument that will be able to detect a meaningful and interpretable treatment benefit in clinical trials, and support approval and labeling claims.

This early assistance can be particularly important for COAs used in clinical trials to develop new therapies for PRD, given the challenges of studying this patient population. The Team has been able to offer creative and flexible advice to work with FDA review divisions and instrument developers to overcome some of these challenges. For example, the Team has worked with OPT and CDER's Division of Gastroenterology and Inborn Errors Products (DGIEP) to facilitate COA development for pediatric Crohn's disease by evaluating the existing disease activity index used in pediatric Crohn's disease trials based on the criteria described within the guidance document *Patient-Reported Outcome Measures: Use in Medical Product Development to Support Labeling Claims*. In addition, OPT worked with the Team and DGIEP to systemically review the COAs used in pediatric ulcerative colitis registration trials and published the review findings in 2014 (see Section 3.4.1.2).

3.5.1.3. Strategy: Facilitate Increasing the Knowledge of Biomarkers and Clinical Outcome Assessments Useful for PRD, Including Engaging with Investigators and Organizations in Biomarker and Clinical Outcome Qualification Programs to Advise during Their Development

A biomarker is a characteristic that is objectively measured and evaluated as an indicator of normal biologic processes, pathologic processes, or biological responses to a therapeutic intervention.[43] These measured characteristics can be physiologic, pathologic, or anatomic and can be used as a basis for the selection of patients for inclusion in a clinical trial. Additionally, changes in biomarker measurements following a therapeutic intervention may be used to predict or identify an issue with the safety of the therapy, or an eventual benefit. Using biomarkers to classify patients by disease type or response probability can improve the drug development process by decreasing variability between patients and increasing the treatment effect size.

A COA is a measure of a patient's symptoms, overall mental state, or the effects of a disease on how a patient feels. COAs can be used to determine whether or not a drug has been demonstrated to provide treatment benefit. The elements of a COA are:

- A measure that produces a score, along with clearly defined instructions for administering the COA and assessing the response;

- A standard format for collecting the data; and
- A well-documented methodology for scoring, analysis, and interpretation of the results in the targeted patient population.

There are four types of COAs. Three are distinguished by who is reporting the outcome (i.e., patient, clinician, or observer). The fourth is an assessment of performance (i.e., performance outcome measures).

Expanding the list of available biomarkers and COAs, including those that have formal qualification for use in PRD drug development, is chiefly accomplished by investigators, sponsors, and other organizations outside of FDA; however, FDA's advice can help ensure that their efforts include attention to the aspects that are important to applying the biomarkers and COAs in drug development programs. Further, ongoing and new collaborations of FDA with these organizations can be valuable to increase the availability of biomarkers and COAs. For example, OPT and the part-time Oak Ridge Institute for Science and Education (ORISE) neonatologist are working with CDER's Division of Cardio-Renal Products and external academic scientists to explore the possibility of identifying feasible biomarkers for use in pulmonary arterial hypertension trials in neonates, infants and young children and in PRD, FDA is working with external stakeholders to further develop the use of dystrophin as a biomarker for use in clinical trials of children with Duchenne muscular dystrophy.

One pathway for FDA collaboration is within the Biomarker and COA Qualification Programs that have been established at FDA, as described on FDA's website and the final guidance document, *Qualification Process for Drug Development Tools*. Biomarkers and COAs are two types of drug development tools (DDT) and are part of FDA's Drug Development Tools (DDT) Qualification Programs.[44] While qualification is not necessary to use a biomarker or a COA in development of a drug, qualification is intended to make more biomarkers and COAs well established for their full utility, and sooner than without qualification.

Qualification is a conclusion that within the stated context of use[45], the DDT can be relied upon to have a specific interpretation and application in drug development and regulatory review. Qualification may contribute to acceptance and application of DDTs across multiple drug development programs and having qualified DDTs that can be used by many sponsors will aid in optimizing drug development and evaluation.

In addition, qualified biomarkers and clinical outcome assessments relevant to PRD would improve the understanding of how to develop drugs for these diseases and can therefore stimulate further study of, and drug development for, these diseases. Biomarkers, with their usefulness in identifying patients for inclusion in clinical trials and who are more likely to have a larger treatment effect, can be beneficial in overcoming the issues of small populations for study and heterogeneity. COAs can be used to incorporate clinically meaningful endpoints that are meaningful to patients and are sensitive to showing drug effects, in clinical trials. Having these qualified tools will streamline the development process.

3.5.1.4. Strategy: Develop Training Programs for Pediatric Clinical Investigators

Clinical trials involving children have special scientific, clinical, and ethical considerations. Further, differences in treatment effects between pediatric subpopulations related to age and maturation must be considered. Helping investigators to understand these issues and the regulatory framework within which clinical trials involving children must be performed should help to increase quality investigations in children, including those with rare diseases.

OPT and CDER's PMHS will be conducting a pediatric clinical investigator training session in September 2014, and annually if determined to be needed, in designing and conducting clinical trials in pediatric patients. The course will focus on providing investigators with an understanding of the challenges of studying products in the pediatric population, an overview of extrapolation, a summary of FDA processes and timelines, and an overview of ethically appropriate methods related to the design of clinical trials in the pediatric population. Issues related to orphan product development and network collaborations will also be discussed.

3.5.1.5. Strategy: Explore Modeling and Simulation Approaches (E.G., Physiologically-Based Pharmacokinetic (PBPK) Models) to Provide Preliminary Data for Drugs Used In Pediatric Rare Diseases (PRD) to Inform the Design and Conduct of PK/PD Studies and Other Clinical Trials for Investigational Drugs in PRD Populations

The National Center for Toxicological Research (NCTR) has conducted several studies in collaboration with colleagues at CDER studying the neurotoxicity associated with general anesthetics and sedatives that are often used in pediatric populations. Studies have ranged from in vitro rat models to whole juvenile animal models, including rats and nonhuman primates. This on-going collaboration between NCTR and CDER can be extended to include PRD.

NCTR has developed PBPK models (i.e., computer simulation methods) to explore the design and conduct of PK/PD studies for investigational drugs in pediatric populations. For example, the development of a PBPK model that integrates drug-dependent parameters (e.g., renal clearance, metabolic pathways) and system-dependent parameters (e.g., non-drug parameters such as blood flow rate, protein binding, and enzyme and transporter activities) is one possible approach. Among other uses, this approach may be useful for planning a first-in-pediatric PK study and recommending starting doses for clinical trials. These efforts may be particularly helpful in PRD where available data is limited by small populations.

In addition, considerable work on computational approaches to modeling and simulation in pediatric patients is already ongoing as a collaborative effort of FDA pediatric groups (from OPT, PMHS and the Pediatric Clinical Pharmacology Staff) with the Division of Pharmacometrics in the Office of Clinical Pharmacology in CDER.

NCTR and CDER's Office of Clinical Pharmacology will have further discussions to explore the possibility of collaborating on modeling and simulation efforts to inform studies in PRD. These PRD models might cover pre-clinical studies to clinical drug development to post-marketing assessment of drug safety. Techniques involved may include the development of physiologically-based PK (PBPK) models, traditional non-compartmental models, and combinations of these approaches.

3.5.2. Devices

3.5.2.1. Strategy: Develop Expedited Approval Pathway for Certain Devices Intended to Treat Unmet Medical Needs

FDA is proposing a voluntary expedited access PMA program for certain medical devices which demonstrate the potential to address unmet medical needs[46] for life threatening or irreversibly debilitating diseases or conditions. This program should further expedite the development, assessment and review of these important medical devices, in order to have earlier access to fulfill an unmet need, including for rare pediatric diseases. Expedited Access PMA (EAP) Devices (i.e., devices that qualify for the EAP program) must meet the statutory standard of PMA approval of reasonable assurance of safety and effectiveness.[47]

Under this program the basis for PMA approval may rely on assessments of a device's effect on an intermediate or surrogate endpoint[48] that is reasonably likely to predict clinical benefit (on the condition that the remaining uncertainty about the predictive relationship between a surrogate and clinical benefit is minimized through confirmatory post-approval studies or on the condition that clinical benefit is verified through confirmatory post-approval studies).

Since EAP Devices demonstrate the potential to address unmet medical needs for life threatening or irreversibly debilitating diseases or conditions, in order to help patients have more timely access to these medical devices, FDA may accept less certainty regarding the benefit-risk profile of these devices at the time of premarket approval, and approve an EAP Device, as long as the data still support a reasonable assurance of safety and effectiveness. That is, FDA intends to approve an EAP Device if the uncertainty is sufficiently balanced by other factors, including the probable benefits of the device, the probable benefits of earlier patient access to the device, and postmarket controls, to support premarket approval.

Other features of EAP include: as resources permit, more interactive communications during device development and more interactive review of IDE applications and PMA applications; involvement of, where appropriate, Office and Center-level senior management and experienced review staff in a proactive, collaborative, cross-disciplinary review; where appropriate, and resources permitting, assignment of a cross-disciplinary case manager; and priority review[49].

In addition, as part of the EAP program, on a case-by-case basis, FDA may, where appropriate, allow a sponsor to provide less manufacturing information in their PMA application. Note, a device must be in conformance with the Quality System (QS) regulation (QSReg) and the sponsor must submit adequate information in the PMA to meet the requirements under section 515(c)(1)(C) of the FD&C Act and 21 CFR 814.20(b)(4)(v). In appropriate cases, FDA may also, at its discretion, conduct certain manufacturing inspections after product approval. Where an inspection is not conducted prior to approval of the PMA application for an EAP Device, FDA intends to conduct an inspection within twelve months after approval.

A draft guidance document titled *Expedited Access for Premarket Approval Medical Devices Intended for Unmet Medical Need for Life Threatening or Irreversibly Debilitating Diseases or Conditions* was issued on April 23, 2014, for comment purposes and may be consulted for further details on the program.

3.5.2.2. Strategy: Evaluate the Results of an Analysis of Approved Medical Devices to Explore the Feasibility of Shifting Some Premarket Data Requirements to the Postmarket Setting for Future Medical Devices

The right balance of premarket and postmarket data collection facilitates timely patient access to important new technologies for PRD patients, without undermining patient safety. At the time of device approval, certain safety and effectiveness questions may not be fully resolved. This can be due to significant obstacles, such as the time and cost involved addressing possible rare adverse events or longterm safety issues. Further, controlled clinical studies do not fully represent the benefit-risk profile of a device when used in real-world clinical practice.

FDA has long applied postmarket controls as a way to reduce premarket data collection, where appropriate, while assuring that the statutory standard for approval of reasonable assurance of safety and effectiveness is still met. Section 513(a)(3)(C) of the FD&C Act specifically requires FDA to consider the use of postmarket controls in lieu of collecting and reviewing all effectiveness data prior to PMA approval. While this shift of some premarket data to the postmarket setting has the potential to directly impact patient access to high-quality, safe, and effective medical devices of public health importance, there are conditions which must be fulfilled. Adequate assurances that necessary and timely data collection will occur and capabilities to quickly remove the device from the market if postmarket data does not support reasonable assurances of safety and effectiveness, or is not provided in a reasonable timeframe, must be available.

A draft guidance document titled *Balancing Premarket and Postmarket Data Collection for Devices Subject to Premarket Approval* was issued on April 23, 2014, for comment purposes only and may be consulted for further details.

In order to help further assure the appropriate balance between premarket and postmarket data requirements is assessed for all patients, including PRD patients, CDRH is conducting an analysis of device types subject to a PMA that have been on the market, in order to determine whether or not to shift some premarket data requirements to the postmarket setting, or to pursue down classification. Interpretation of this analysis will support efforts in striking the right balance between premarket and postmarket data requirements, with the possible benefits of earlier patient access to certain devices, particularly when the alternatives are either absent or of limited use. With regard to rare pediatric diseases, this is particularly important, due to the challenges of obtaining clinical data in this patient population.

3.5.2.3. Strategy: Support the Development of Medical Device Development to Improve Clinical Trial Performance

CDRH published a draft guidance document, *Medical Device Development Tools*, describing how medical device development tools can be validated and accepted by the Center as clinical endpoints for premarket medical device studies. In addition to COAs and Biomarker Tests, CDRH also describes a pathway for Nonclinical Assessment Models (NAM). These are nonclinical test methods or models to reflect device function or in vivo performance. A NAM can be an in vitro test, animal, or computational model. The use of these medical device development tools can streamline the preclinical phase of device development.

3.5.2.4. Strategy: Develop Curriculum for Undergraduate/Graduate Studies to Increase Understanding of Regulatory Approval Process for Device Development

CDRH is creating a curriculum to be used in undergraduate and graduate studies to help inventors, engineers, entrepreneurs and innovators better understand the regulatory approval process. One of the case studies involves getting devices for pediatric populations to the market. This early education will help improve the efficiency of the development process, including the development of devices for children with rare diseases.

3.5.3. General

3.5.3.1. Strategy: Use FDA Web-Based Resources to Update and Expand Awareness of PRD Product Development Issues

Web-based resources are becoming increasingly more important as tools for education and for navigating complex processes. Two web-based resources have recently been launched to support rare disease drug development, including pediatrics. Use of these resources will serve to increase their value in the development of products for rare diseases.

CDER's RDP, in collaboration with NIH, has developed an internet-based navigational tool[50] designed to enable investigator-initiated IND application submissions. It was primarily developed to support rare disease drug development and is intended for a broad audience of academic investigators, small pharmaceutical businesses, and anyone searching for brief explanations about various aspects of IND application submissions and procedures.

OPT has developed a web page which provides practitioners, caregivers, and researchers with the following information: a brief summary of new pediatric labeling information for the last 500-plus products studied in pediatrics; a link to the reviews that were performed on the submitted pediatric studies; a link to the outcomes and list of products that have been reviewed for postmarketing safety by the Pediatric Advisory Committee; a link to the publications that FDA has produced analyzing the pediatric studies submitted; and a link to ethical issues and presentations on pediatric ethics topics.

OOPD has developed an educational resource for patients, advocacy groups, investigators, and orphan product developers.[51] This resource page provides links to recorded sessions on cross-cutting rare disease topics such as the essentials of interacting with FDA, a workshop on natural history studies in rare diseases, and a course in the science of small clinical trials. Topics will continue to be added to the site.

OOPD also plans to develop a web-based rare disease portal, as an entry portal for stakeholders to more easily link to the relevant FDA sites for information and guidance on regulatory issues and available programs.

3.5.3.2. Strategy: Increase Awareness in Pediatric Rare Disease Researchers, Product Developers, and Patient Community of Funding Opportunities through OPD Grant Program

The OPD grant program has an annual budget of approximately $14 million to fund clinical development of drugs, biological products, medical devices, and medical foods for rare diseases. OOPD will further increase the awareness in the pediatric community of these funding opportunities through outreach and other collaborations.

3.6. Objective 4: Enhance FDA Review Process for PRD Products

3.6.1. Drugs/Biologics

3.6.1.1. Strategy: Foster FDA's Efforts to Obtain Patients' and Caregivers' Perspectives for Incorporation in Drug Development

Patient participation in the process of drug development is important because only they can provide the unique perspective on their disease, its impact on daily life, and the tolerability of currently available therapies. Through an understanding of the patients' or their caregivers' perspectives, developers can assure that potential treatment effects on aspects of daily life that are important to patients are adequately captured in clinical trials. These perspectives can also be used to develop COAs that are meaningful to patients and their caregivers, and information on tolerability of currently available therapies can be useful in identifying unmet medical needs. Further, this information can be helpful to FDA's review of applications for new drugs, particularly when the impact of a disease on patients is not well understood or endpoints for studying drugs for a disease are not clearly defined or established.

The Patient Focused Drug Development Program provides a mechanism for obtaining patients' and caregivers input on specific disease areas, and FDA has committed to 20 disease areas over five years. Considerations in the selection process included disease areas:

- That are chronic, symptomatic, or affect functioning and activities of daily living;
- For which aspects of the disease are not formally captured in clinical trials; and
- For which there are currently no therapies or very few therapies, or the available therapies do not directly affect how a patient feels or functions.

For each disease area selected, the agency is conducting a public meeting to discuss the disease and its impact on patients' daily lives, the types of treatment benefits that matter most to patients, and patients' and caregivers' perspectives on the adequacy of available therapies. These meetings include participation of FDA review divisions, the relevant patient community, and other interested stakeholders. On June 10, 2014, FDA conducted a meeting on the neurological manifestations of inborn errors of metabolism to hear patients' and caregivers' perspectives of what matters most to them. The Agency may also consider the inclusion of additional pediatric rare disease topics in the selection process for meetings in 2016.

Following each meeting, FDA continues to collect written submissions in the public docket for an additional 60 days. Once the docket closes, those comments are analyzed along with the meeting transcript and webcast comments. This analysis leads to a summary report of the meeting called the 'Voice of the Patient' report. This report is a detailed account that documents, in the patients' own words, what matters most to them in terms of impacts of the disease and treatment approaches. These reports serve an important function in communicating to both FDA review staff and the regulated industry what improvements patients would most like to see in their daily lives. FDA believes that the long-term impact of this program will be a better, more informed understanding of how we might find ways to develop new treatments for these and other diseases.

In addition to Patient-Focused Drug Development, FDA frequently engages with the PRD community. Some recent examples include:

- A public meeting held on September 10, 2013 on the drug development process and the importance of the patient's voice that included advocates from the PRD community including caregivers of children suffering from Mucopolysaccharidoses (MPS);
- A meeting with caregivers and investigators about clinical trial designs for Niemann-Pick Type C disease, held at the 2013 annual conference of the National Niemann-Pick Disease Foundation; and
- Collaborating with a coalition of stakeholders on draft guidance to help accelerate development and review of potential therapies for Duchenne muscular dystrophy.

In addition, in February 2015, FDA is holding a stakeholders meeting to review progress made in development of pediatric therapies. This meeting will be used to inform the Report to Congress that is due by July 2016 on Pediatric Product Development.

The Patient Representative Program provides FDA with the unique perspective of patients and family members affected by a serious or life-threatening disease. Patient representatives can serve in several ways, including as participants on Advisory Committees, as consultants for review divisions, and as presenters at FDA meetings and workshops on disease-specific or regulatory and health policy issues. FDA is committed to ensuring that rare disease patients and caregivers have an opportunity to serve as Patient Representatives, and often partners with rare disease patient advocacy organizations to identify qualified individuals to recruit for the program.

To further ensure patient participation in the product development process, section 1137 of FDASIA requires that FDA "develop and implement strategies to solicit the views of patients during the medical product development process and consider the perspectives of patients during regulatory discussions, including by—(1) fostering participation of a patient representative who may serve as a special government employee in appropriate agency meetings with medical product sponsors and investigators; and (2) exploring means to provide for identification of patient representatives who do not have any, or have minimal, financial interests in the medical products industry."

OHCA is responsible for implementing section 1137, and has established an agency-wide workgroup consisting of key staff members to develop strategies and facilitate implementation activities for including patients' perspectives in regulatory decision-making. These strategies and implementation plans will be articulated in an agency-wide procedures document.

The workgroup is planning to solicit public comment on potential strategies under section 1137, including input from the PRD patient community.

3.6.1.2. Strategy: Further Develop and Implement a Structured Approach to Benefit-Risk Assessment in the Drug Review Process

The benefit-risk assessment in drug review is critical to PRD patients. As an area of further development, FDA has been developing a structured approach to the benefit-risk assessment, in addition to exploring approaches to evaluating and communicating the uncertainty in the Agency's assessment of benefit and risk. FDA's regulatory decisions are informed by an extensive body of evidence on a drug's safety and efficacy. In many cases, this evidence is subject to uncertainty arising from many sources. For example, there is the uncertainty in the degree to which premarket clinical trial data translates to the postmarket setting, when the drug is exposed to a wider patient population. Drawing conclusions in the face of uncertainty can be complex and challenging, and being explicit about the impact of uncertainty on decision-making is an important part of communicating regulatory decisions.

FDA plans to implement a benefit-risk framework in the review of marketing applications for new drug and biologic products, including such applications for pediatric rare diseases. A structured approach to benefit-risk assessment in the review process will enable better communication of the reasoning behind regulatory decisions and ensure, on a more consistent basis, that these decisions are made in an established context that includes an understanding of the severity of the treated condition and the adequacy of the available therapies.

In the area of PRD, consideration of the context of the regulatory decision is particularly important since it helps shape how FDA weighs any safety concerns against the benefits of the new product demonstrated in clinical studies. For rare serious diseases, FDA understands that a patient or caregivers may have a high tolerance for the risk associated with a given therapy. This perspective is a critical element of FDA's decision-making and oversight of the drug development process. It is acknowledged by FDA's Patient Focused Drug Development Initiative that seeks to better understand perspectives on disease severity and current treatment options for certain diseases over the next several years. This information can greatly inform FDA's benefit-risk assessment. The consistent application of a structured approach to benefit-risk assessment should facilitate continuation of FDA's flexibility and innovation in the review and approval of drugs for this patient population.

3.6.1.3. Strategy: Issue Rare Pediatric Disease PRV Draft Guidance Document

The Rare Pediatric Disease PRV is a new incentive program under FDASIA to promote the development of drugs for rare pediatric diseases. Under this program, if a sponsor develops a new drug for the treatment of a rare pediatric disease, when that drug is approved for that disease and if the criteria of the FDASIA provision are met, the sponsor is eligible to receive a voucher that can be redeemed for priority review of another drug application that would not otherwise be eligible. The issuance of a draft guidance document will provide advice to sponsors, further clarify the eligibility criteria for the voucher program, and allow an opportunity for public comments to be submitted for the agency to consider in developing a final guidance document.

3.6.1.4. Strategy: Continue Reviewer Training for Rare Diseases and PRD

FDA has developed education and annual training programs for FDA reviewers related to development, review, and approval of drugs for rare diseases. This training helps to familiarize reviewers with the challenges associated with rare disease applications, including applications for drugs to treat PRD, and the strategies to address those challenges. It encourages flexibility and scientific judgment in the review and regulation of rare disease applications. The program provides additional training to reviewers on applying FDA's expedited programs (e.g., fast track, accelerated approval, priority review, and breakthrough therapy) to rare disease product development programs, including PRD, and helps ensure these programs are utilized to their fullest extent. Both OPT and PMHS have provided training specifically relating to PRD in previous years. In addition, the Agency will include a standing pediatric representative on the planning committee for these meetings. Continuing these reviewer training programs will help promote increased consistency of scientific and regulatory approaches across applications and review teams.

3.6.1.5. Strategy: Explore Potential for Innovation in Data Analysis

Clinical trials for PRD treatments are usually of small size and as a result, face challenges in the ability to support inference about experimental therapies. A common solution often proposed is to conduct a single-arm study, without the use of randomization or a concurrent control group, which may cause difficulties in interpreting the study's results.

Exploring the potential for innovation in data analysis for PRD may help to overcome some of these challenges and further development of therapies for them. FDA is also investigating ways to encourage sponsors contemplating innovative approaches, including PRD sponsors, to meet with FDA and discuss their options early in study planning. Examples of innovative approaches may include Bayesian methods to incorporate historical/external data, Bayesian hierarchical modeling of rare disease subtypes, and structured meta-analyses assessments to explore safety issues and risks.

3.6.2. Devices

3.6.2.1. Strategy: Further Develop Methods to Implement the Incorporation of Patient Preferences into Assessments of Premarket Approval and De Novo Classifications of Devices

Similar to the initiatives to incorporate patient preferences into the development and review of drug products, the Patient Preference Initiative was created to better incorporate the voice of patients on the benefit-risk trade-offs of medical devices into the full spectrum of regulatory decision making. It also aims to advance the science of measuring treatment preferences of patients, caregivers, and health care providers, and incorporate this information into the Medical Device Total Product Life Cycle (TPLC) regulatory paradigm.

It began with a series of meetings sponsored by NORD and it led to a variety of additional efforts that are relevant to PRD patients. In 2012, a guidance document, *Factors to Consider When Making Benefit-Risk Determinations in Medical Device Premarket Approval and De Novo Classifications*, was published that created a systematic patient-centric benefit-risk framework, which includes a template for reviewers to further assure decisions are consistent across premarket submissions. In September 2013, a workshop was held to further explore methods of incorporating patient preferences into the TPLC.

Additionally, one of the projects of the MDIC is to determine the availability of regulatory science tools for measuring patient preferences in a properly validated method that could be used by FDA, and incorporated into the benefit-risk framework.

Advancing these methods to incorporate patient preferences into medical device development and regulatory decision making will benefit children with rare diseases through a better understanding of their unmet needs and will facilitate getting products to the market to serve them.

3.6.2.2. Strategy: Establish a Patient Engagement Panel as Part of CDRH's Medical Advisory Committee

CDRH will establish a Patient Engagement Panel as part of its Medical Device Advisory Committee to serve as a body of experts to provide feedback, advice, and recommendations to FDA on cross-cutting issues such as patient related outcomes, medical device labeling, and the use of medical devices at home. This strategy will assist in getting needed medical devices to the market for children with rare diseases.

3.6.2.3. Strategy: Analyze the HDE Process for Medical Devices That Diagnose and Treat PRD

OOPD and CDRH are conducting an analysis of HDE applications to determine the reasons they were deemed approvable or not. This information will be useful to give better advice to sponsors of devices for rare diseases. The analysis will include also a pediatric sub-focus to specifically benefit the development of devices for this population.

Other analyses of the pediatric HDEs will consider certain pediatric HDE approval requirements: All pediatric HDE applications that include a request for a waiver of the profit-making restriction are reviewed annually by the Pediatric Advisory Committee as to the product's safety and ongoing appropriateness. If the risk-benefit balance between the need for the product and its safety profile has shifted, the product will be referred back to CDRH for additional assessment.

3.6.2.4. Strategy: Set Standards for Whole Genome Sequencing That Can Be Used as a Comparator

There are several different genetic testing methods that have recently been cleared for specific diagnostic tests. These clearances outline a pathway to market for genetic testing to include diagnosis of rare genetic pediatric diseases. These include diagnostic arrays and next gen sequencing. FDA is currently working with the National Institute of Standards and Technology on standards for whole genome sequencing that can be used as a comparator. This will help to further genetic testing, including testing for PRD.

3.6.3. General

3.6.3.1. Strategy: Continue to Enhance FDA's Expertise to Review Innovative Products

As science expands and continues to drive the development of innovative therapies, continuing to build upon FDA's expertise and capacity to review these innovative products will help make products for the treatment of children with rare diseases more available.

For example, FDA is considering outlining the requirements for a third party or end user to 3-D print medical devices outside a traditional manufacturing setting. Outlining these requirements will also help the Agency's PDC to better guide pediatric innovators of products such as the pediatric 3-D artificial trachea that was assisted in part by the PDC. Additionally, FDA recognizes the need for more individuals to be appropriately trained in the evaluation of regulatory evidence. The emerging field of regulatory science involves the application of scientific methods to improve the development, review and oversight of new drugs, biologics, devices and food products that require regulatory approval.

FDA is one of the premier agencies for regulatory research and training in the United States, and as such has created a number of strong training programs for its staff including the Staff Colleges within each Center which offer numerous courses covering a range of regulatory, scientific and professional development topics. Also, the agency administers several professional development programs, including the IPA Program with academic institutions, the ORISE fellowships, and the Commissioner's Fellowship Program. In 2013, FDA was able to utilize the ORISE program to support a part-time two year fellowship for a senior neonatologist to help advance the Agency's efforts to support product development in neonates. Neonatology is an area Congress has targeted for further development and FDA plans to recruit the expertise necessary to further this initiative.

Further, in support of FDA's Advancing Regulatory Science Initiative, FDA is working with a number of external stakeholders to introduce the concept of a consortium model to develop a robust regulatory science education and training platform to prepare future regulatory scientists working in government, academia, industry and the non-profit arena. The goal for a consortium concept is not to duplicate content that is currently available in the academic setting. It is to supplement existing academic programs, filling the gaps which are known to exist in traditional educational programs and training modules that do not access, nor fully understand, the range of regulatory content that is available.

Noted above are examples of ways in which FDA is promoting education and training in regulatory science. Continuing to build on these efforts will help increase the availability of new therapies for all patients, including children with rare diseases.

3.7. Conclusion

There are many challenges to developing new therapies for PRD. These challenges include the difficulty of conducting clinical trials in small populations affected by diseases whose natural histories are not well characterized, as well as addressing the added safeguards required when involving children in those trials. These are complex issues and most single entities (e.g., medical product manufacturer, academic institution, or governmental agency) generally do not have sufficient resources or expertise to independently develop products to treat PRD efficiently. Therefore, networks, partnerships, and collaborations are crucial to the success of developing new therapies for PRD. Among other benefits, these relationships can facilitate filling foundational science information gaps, as well as the recruitment for, and conduct of, clinical trials. Further, it is important to recognize that patients, families, and advocacy groups have much to contribute throughout the development process.

Additionally, FDA encourages developers of these new therapies to engage with FDA often and early in the development process in order to exchange ideas, discuss appropriate paths forward and obtain advice in navigating the regulatory process.

FDA has many initiatives that can help to meet the goal of accelerating the development of new tests and therapies to diagnose and treat PRD. These initiatives, identified as key strategies, are situated beneath four objectives that cascade from FDA's draft Core Mission Goals and Objectives. The objectives are defined and ordered chronologically based on the product development process. These objectives include enhancing foundational and translational science, strengthening FDA's collaborations within and outside the Agency, advancing the use of regulatory science to aid clinical trial design and performance, and enhancing FDA's review process, all with the focus on PRD.

The strategies beneath the objectives range from those directed specifically at PRD, such as the incentives provided by the Rare Pediatric Disease PRV Program, and identifying unmet pediatric needs in medical device development for rare diseases, to those broader in scope, such as the Drug Development Tools Qualification Program, the Medical Device Development Tools Program (now in draft) and exploring the feasibility of shifting certain premarket data requirements to the postmarket setting, where appropriate, in the approval of medical devices. Enhancing and strengthening these initiatives will serve to further accelerate the development of new therapies for children with rare diseases, as will FDA's continuing to build expertise and capacity to review these innovative products for safety and effectiveness.

Finally, FDA believes the strategies in this document will help to accelerate the development of new therapies to treat PRD by increasing stakeholders' awareness of the many FDA programs and initiatives to facilitate the development process.

APPENDICES

Appendix 1: DRAFT FDA Core Mission Goals and Objectives

As discussed in the Report, the Strategic Plan Objectives are linked to and support the DRAFT FDA Core Mission Goals and Objectives (See Appendix 2 for Crosswalk the Strategic Plan Objectives with FDA's Core Mission Objectives),

---

1. Enhance oversight of FDA-regulated products

1.1 Increase the use of regulatory science to inform standards development, analysis and decision-making

1.2 Reduce risks in the manufacturing, production, and distribution of FDA-regulated products

1.3 Strengthen detection and surveillance of problems with FDA-regulated products

1.4 Improve response to identified and emerging problems with FDA-regulated products

---

2. Improve and safeguard access to FDA-regulated products to benefit health

2.1 Increase regulatory science capacity to effectively evaluate products

2.2 Improve the effectiveness of the product development process

2.3 Improve the predictability, consistency, transparency, and efficiency of the review process

3. Promote better informed decisions about the use of FDA-regulated products

3.1 Strengthen social and behavioral science to help patients, consumers and professionals make informed decisions about regulated products

3.2 Improve patient and providers access to benefit-risk information about FDA-regulated products

3.3 Improve safety and health information provided to the public

4. Strengthen organizational excellence and accountability

4.1 Recruit, develop, retain and strategically manage a world-class workforce 4.2 Improve the overall operation and effectiveness of FDA

4.3 Invest in infrastructure to enhance productivity and capabilities

Source: "Office of the Commissioner; Request for Comments on the Food and Drug Administration Fiscal Year 2014-2018 Strategic Priorities Document; Request for Comments" 79 Federal Register 126 (1 July 2014), pp. 37332-37333.

APPENDIX 2: CROSSWALK BETWEEN THE STRATEGIC PLAN AND FDA CORE MISSION OBJECTIVES

1. Enhance foundational and translational science for PRD

2.1. Increase regulatory science capacity to effectively evaluate products

2.2. Improve the effectiveness of the product development process

2. Strengthen communication, collaboration and partnering for PRD within and outside FDA

2.2. Improve the effectiveness of the product development process

2.3. Improve the predictability, consistency, transparency, and efficiency of the review process

3.1. Improve patient and providers access to benefit-risk information about FDA-regulated products

4.2. Improve the overall operation and effectiveness of FDA

3. Advance the use of regulatory science for PRD to aid clinical trial design and performance

1.1. Increase the use of regulatory science to inform standards development, analysis and decision-making

2.1. Increase regulatory science capacity to effectively evaluate products

2.2. Improve the effectiveness of the product development process

4. Enhance FDA review process for PRD products

2.3. Improve the predictability, consistency, transparency, and efficiency of the review process

3.1. Improve patient and providers access to benefit-risk information about FDA-regulated products

4.2. Improve the overall operation and effectiveness of FDA

APPENDIX 3: PUBLIC WORKSHOP SPEAKERS AND PANELISTS

Complex Issues in Developing Drug and Biological
Products for Rare Diseases

January 6, 2014

*Alphabetically ordered by last name

- Nuria Carrillo-Carrasco, M.D., Division of Preclinical Innovation, National Center for Advancing Translational Sciences (NCATS), National Institutes of Health (NIH)
- Edward M. Cox, M.D., M.P.H., Director, Office of Antimicrobial Products, Center for Drug Evaluation and Research (CDER), FDA
- Diane Edquist Dorman, Vice President, Public Policy, National Organization for Rare Disorders (NORD)
- Stephen C. Groft, Pharm.D., Director, Office of Rare Diseases Research, NCATS, NIH
- Nicole Mayer Hamblett, Ph.D., Associate Professor, Pediatrics, Adjunct Associate Professor, Biostatistics, University of Washington; Co-Director, Cystic Fibrosis Therapeutics Development Network

Coordinating Center; Director, Seattle Children's Core for Biomedical Statistics, Seattle Children's Research Institute

- John Hyde, Ph.D., M.D., Medical Officer, Division of Clinical Evaluation and Pharmacology/Toxicology, Office of Cellular, Tissue and Gene Therapies (OCTGT), Center for Biologics Evaluation and Research (CBER), FDA
- Emil D. Kakkis, M.D., Ph.D., President and Founder, EveryLife Foundation for Rare Diseases; Chief Executive Officer and President, Ultragenyx Pharmaceutical
- Mwango Kashoki, M.D., M.P.H., Associate Director for Safety, Office of New Drugs (OND), CDER, FDA
- Michael R. Kosorok, Ph.D., M.S., Chair, Department of Biostatistics, Professor, Department of Statistics and Operations Research, University of North Carolina-Chapel Hill
- Robert Kowalski, Pharm.D., Global Head Drug Regulatory Affairs & U.S. Head of Development Novartis Pharmaceuticals Corporation,
- Matthias Kretzler, M.D., Warner-Lambert/Parke-Davis Professor of Medicine/Nephrology, Research Professor in Computational Medicine and Bioinformatics, University of Michigan Medical School
- Sandra L. Kweder, M.D., F.A.C.P., Acting Director, Study Endpoints and Labeling Development (SEALD), Deputy Director, OND, CDER, FDA
- Paul Lasko, Ph.D., Professor, Department of Biology, McGill University, Montréal, Québec, Canada; Chair, International Rare Diseases Research Consortium (IRDiRC)
- John C. McKew, Ph.D., Acting Scientific Director, Division of Preclinical Innovation, NCATS, NIH
- Richard A. Moscicki, M.D., Deputy Center Director for Science Operations, CDER, FDA
- Andrew E. Mulberg, M.D., F.A.A.P, C.P.I. , Deputy Director, Division of Gastroenterology and Inborn Error Products (DGIEP), CDER, FDA
- Anne Pariser, M.D., Associate Director, Rare Disease Program, OND, CDER, FDA
- Ira Shoulson, M.D., Professor of Neurology, Pharmacology and Human Science, Director, Program for Regulatory Science & Medicine, Georgetown University
- Marshall L. Summar, M.D., Chief, Genetics and Metabolism, Children's National Medical Center Washington D.C.

- Ellis F. Unger, M.D., Director, Office of Drug Evaluation-I, CDER, FDA
- Marc K. Walton, M.D., Ph.D., Associate Director, Office of Translational Sciences, CDER, FDA
- Pamela M. Williamson, R.A.C., F.R.A.P.S., Senior Vice President and Global Head, Regulatory Affairs & Compliance, Genzyme; Representative for Biotechnology Industry Organization (BIO)

Encouraging and Accelerating Development of New Therapies for Pediatric Rare Diseases

January 7, 2014

Alphabetically ordered by last name

- Peter C. Adamson, M.D., Chair, Children's Oncology Group; Professor of Pediatrics and Pharmacology, University of Pennsylvania School of Medicine; Chief, Division of Clinical Pharmacology and Therapeutics, The Children's Hospital of Philadelphia
- David Arons, J.D., Senior Director of Public Policy, National Brain Tumor Society
- Robert J. Beall, Ph.D., President and Chief Executive Officer, Cystic Fibrosis Foundation
- Daniel Benjamin Jr., M.D., Ph.D., M.P.H., Associate Director, Duke Clinical Research Institute, Duke University of School of Medicine
- Amy Celento, Patient Representative, FDA's Pediatric Advisory Committee; National Vice President, The Cooley's Anemia Foundation, Inc.
- Lawrence Charnas, M.D., Ph.D., Director and Head of Discovery Medicine Research, Shire Pharmaceuticals
- Katie Clapp, M.S., President and Executive Director, FRAXA Research Foundation
- Edward Connor, M.D., M.B.E., Children's National Health System and Clinical and Translational Sciences Institute, Children's National Medical Center; Professor of Pediatrics, Microbiology, Immunology, and Tropical Medicine, George Washington School of Medicine and Health Sciences; Co-Director, Innovative Strategies and Services, Clinical and Translational Research Institute at Children's National

- Alejandro Dorenbaum, M.D., Chief Medical Officer, Lumena Pharmaceuticals
- Anne-Virginie Eggimann, M.Sc., bluebird bio, Inc.
- Maryam Fouladi, M.D., M.Sc., Cincinnati Children's Hospital Medical Center
- Patricia Furlong, Founding President and CEO Parent Project Muscular Dystrophy
- Nancy Goodman, Founder and Executive Director, Kids v Cancer
- Holcombe Grier, M.D., Professor of Pediatrics, Harvard Medical School
- Lee Helman, M.D., National Cancer Institute, NIH; Professor of Pediatrics and Oncology, Johns Hopkins University
- Katherine High, M.D., Investigator, Howard Hughes Medical Institute; Director, Center for Cellular and Molecular Therapeutics, The Children's Hospital of Philadelphia
- Steven Hirschfeld, M.D., Ph.D., Eunice Kennedy Shriver National Institute of Child Health and Human Development (NICHD), NIH; Captain, Commissioned Corps, USPHS
- Robert Iannone, M.D., M.S.C.E., Merck and Co., Inc.
- Ilan Irony, M.D., Chief, General Medicine Branch, Division of Clinical Evaluation and Pharmacology/Toxicology, OCTGT, CBER, FDA
- Jessica Lee, M.D., M.M.Sc., Medical Officer, Team Leader, GGIEP, CDER, FDA
- Cynthia Le Mons, Executive Director and CEO, National Urea Cycle Disorders Foundation
- Philip Marella, Niemann-Pick Type C Disease, Trustee, Dana's Angels Research Trust; President, Green Light Worldwide Media, Inc.,
- D. Elizabeth McNeil, M.D., M.Sc., National Institute of Neurological Disorders and Stroke, NIH
- Jana Monaco, Advocacy Liaison, Organic Acidemia Association; Patient/Family Advisory Council Chair at Children's National Medical Center
- Andrew Mulberg, M.D., F.A.A.P., C.P.I., Deputy Director, DGIEP, CDER, FDA
- Dianne Murphy, M.D., F.A.A.P., Director, Office of Pediatric Therapeutics (OPT), FDA
- Robert "Skip" Nelson, M.D., Ph.D., Deputy Director and Senior Pediatric Ethicist, OPT, FDA

- Daniel Ory, M.D., Chair, Scientific Advisory Board, National Niemann-Pick Disease Foundation; Co-Director; Diabetic Cardiovascular Disease Center; Director of Admissions, Division of Biology and Biomedical Sciences; Associate Director of the Medical Scientist Training Program; Director of the Metabolomics Facility, Washington University School of Medicine
- Darrile Papier, Patient Advocate
- Gail Pearson, M.D., Sc.D., F.A.C.C., F.A.H.A., F.A.A.P., Director, Office of Clinical Research, National Heart, Lung, and Blood Institute, NIH
- Holly Peay, M.S., C.G.C., Parent Project Muscular Dystrophy
- Betsy Peterson, Founder, The Children's Heart Foundation
- Forbes Porter, M.D., Ph.D., NICHD, NIH
- Gregory Reaman, M.D., Associate Director of Oncology Sciences, Office of Hematology and Oncology Products, CDER, FDA; Professor of Pediatrics, The George Washington University School of Medicine and Health Sciences
- Lori Sames, CEO and Co-Founder, Hannah's Hope Fund
- Malcolm Smith, M.D., Ph.D., Associate Branch Chief, Pediatrics, Cancer Therapy Evaluation Program, National Cancer Institute (NCI); Program Director, Primary NCI Liaison to Childhood Cancer Investigators, Children's Oncology Group
- Brenda Weigel, M.D., M.Sc., Director, Division of Pediatric Hematology/Oncology, University of Minnesota Amplatz Children's Hospital
- Susan L. Weiner, Ph.D., President and Founder, The Children's Cause for Cancer Advocacy
- David Williams, M.D., Chief, Division of Hematology/Oncology, Director, Translational Research, Boston Children's Hospital (BCH); Associate Chairman, Department of Pediatric Oncology, Dana-Farber Cancer Institute (DFCI); Director, Pediatric Hematology/Oncology Fellowship Training Program, BCH/DFCI
- Anne Willis, MA, Director, Division of Cancer Survivorship, George Washington University Cancer Institute; Director, GW Center for the Advancement of Cancer Survivorship, Navigation and Policy
- Lynne Yao, MD, Associate Director, Pediatric and Maternal Health, OND, CDER, FDA

- Anne Zajicek, M.D., Pharm.D., Chief, Obstetric and Pediatric Pharmacology and Therapeutics Branch, NICHD

Complex Issues in Developing Medical Devices for Pediatric Patients Affected by Rare Diseases

January 8, 2014

- Eric Chen, M.S., Director, Humanitarian Use Devices Program, Office of Orphan Products Development (OOPD), FDA
- Diane Edquist Dorman, Vice President, Public Policy, NORD
- Christy Foreman, M.S., Director, Office of Device Evaluation (ODE), Center for Devices and Radiologic Health (CDRH), FDA
- Jacqueline Francis, M.D., Medical Officer, Division of Surgical Devices, CDRH, FDA
- James Geiger, M.D., Professor of Surgery, Executive Director, Medical Innovation Center, University of Michigan
- Stephen Groft, PharmD, Director, Office of Rare Diseases Research, NCATS, NIH
- Alberto Gutierrez, Ph.D., Director, Office of In Vitro Diagnostics and Radiological Health, CDRH, FDA
- Tamar Haro, Assistant Director, Department of Federal Affairs, American Academy of Pediatrics
- Steven Hirschfeld, M.D., Ph.D., NICHD, NIH; Captain, Commissioned Corps, USPHS
- John Laschinger, M.D., Medical Officer, Division of Cardiovascular Devices, CDRH, FDA
- Debra Lewis, OD, MBA, Deputy Director, OOPD, FDA
- Markham Luke, M.D., Ph.D., Deputy Director, ODE, CDRH, FDA
- Michelle McMurry-Heath, M.D., Ph.D., Associate Director for Science, CDRH, FDA
- Michael C. Morton, Vice President for Global Regulatory Affairs, Medtronic, Inc.
- Robert "Skip" Nelson, M.D., Ph.D., Deputy Director and Senior Pediatric Ethicist, OPT, FDA
- Gayatri R. Rao, M.D., J.D., Director, OOPD, FDA
- Jacqueline Ryan, M.D., Medical Officer, Division of Anesthesia, General Hospital, Infection Control and Dental Devices, CDRH, FDA

- Murray Sheldon, M.D., Associate Director for Technology and Innovation, CDRH, FDA
- Laura Thompson, Ph.D., Division of Biostatistics, CDRH, FDA
- Linda Ulrich, M.D., Director, Pediatric Device Consortia Grant Program, OOPD, FDA
- Victoria Wagman, Health Scientist, Office of the Center Director, CDRH
- Nicole Wolanski, Captain, USPHS, Director, Premarket Approval Section, ODE, CDRH, FDA

End Notes

[1] Food and Drug Administration Safety and Innovation Act, 2012 PL 112–144 (July 9, 2012).

[2] As set forth in Section 510 of FDASIA Pediatric Rare Diseases, a public meeting shall be held, not later than 18 months after the date of enactment of the Act; and a report including a strategic plan for encouraging and accelerating the development of new therapies for treating pediatric rare diseases shall be issued, not later than 180 days after the date of the public meeting.

[3] The Prescription Drug User Fee Act Reauthorization Performance Goals and Procedures Fiscal Years 2013 through FY 2017 Section IX.E.4. states FDA's agreement that by mid-FY 2014, FDA, through the Rare Disease Program, will conduct a public meeting to discuss complex issues in clinical trials for studying drugs for rare diseases, including such questions as endpoint selection, use of surrogate endpoints/Accelerated Approval, and clinical significance of primary endpoints; reasonable safety exposures; assessment of dose selection; and development of patient-reported outcome instruments. Participants in the discussion will include FDA staff, academic and clinical experts, and industry experts. A summary from the meeting will be made available publicly through the FDA website.

[4] Public Law 112–144 (July 9, 2012).

[5] Public Law 98-551 (October 30, 1984).

[6] Public Law 97-414 (January 4, 1983).

[7] 21 USC 360bb(2): [T] the term "rare disease or condition" means any disease or condition which (A) affects less than 200,000 persons in the United States, or (B) affects more than 200,000 in the United States and for which there is no reasonable expectation that the cost of developing and making available in the United States a drug for such disease or condition will be recovered from sales in the United States of such drug. Determinations under the preceding sentence with respect to any drug shall be made on the basis of the facts and circumstances as of the date the request for designation of the drug under this subsection is made.

[8] http://report.nih.gov/NIHfactsheets/ViewFactSheet.aspx?csid=126&key=R#R

[9] Institute of Medicine. (2010). Rare Diseases and Orphan Products: Accelerating Research and Development.

[10] Pariser, AR, Yao, LP. "Rare Diseases and Orphan Drugs." In *Pediatric Drug Development: Concepts and Applications*, edited by Mulberg AE, et al., Hoboken: John Wiley & Sons Ltd, 2013, http://books.google.com.

[11] Medical foods and dietary supplements are not in the scope of the current therapies, meetings, report, or strategic plan.

[12] "Pediatric" is defined differently in the FD&C Act for drugs (including biological products) and devices. Various regulations and guidance documents address drugs and devices for pediatric indications.

For drugs, 21 CFR 201.57(c)(9)(iv) applies: "From birth to 16 years, including age groups often called neonates, infants, children, and adolescents".

For devices, the Pediatric Medical Device Safety and Improvement Act of 2007, section 303 (a)(6)(E)(i) applies: "The term 'pediatric patients' means patients who are 21 years of age or younger at the time of the diagnosis or treatment"

Section 529 of the FD&C Act Rare Pediatric Disease Priority Review Vouchers defines Rare Pediatric Disease as "the disease primarily affects individuals aged from birth to 18 years, including age groups often called neonates, infants, children, and adolescents."

[13] Institute of Medicine. (2010). Rare Diseases and Orphan Products: Accelerating Research and Development.

[14] Connor EM, Smoyer WE, Davis JM, Zajicek A, Ulrich L, Purucker M, Hirschfeld S. Meeting the Demand for Pediatric Clinical Trials. Sci Transl Med. 2014;6 (227):227fs11.

[15] Public Law 101-629 (November 28, 1990).

[16] A HUD is a medical device intended to benefit patients in the treatment or diagnosis of a disease or condition that affects or is manifested in fewer than 4,000 individuals in the United States per year.

[17]   http://www.fda.gov/MedicalDevices/ProductsandMedicalProcedures/DeviceApprovalsand Clearances/HDEApprovals/ucm161 827.htm

[18] In some cases several of these approaches can be used together to develop a product and get it to market. In 2011, FDA approved the EXCOR Pediatric Ventricular Assist Device, a blood pump that is designed to assist patients whose heart cannot pump enough blood. This product received HUD designation and used OPD Grants program funding to conduct the study used to support approval.

[19] Public Law 107-109 (January 4, 2002).

[20] The BPCA provisions were first enacted in the Better Pharmaceuticals for Children Act as part of the FDA Modernization Act of 1997 (FDAMA, P.L. 105-115).

[21] Public Law 108-155 (December 3, 2003).

[22] Momper, JD, Burckart GJ, Jadhav P. "Applications of Population Pharmacokinetics for Pediatric Drug Development." In *Pediatric Drug Development: Concepts and Applications*, edited by Mulberg AE, et al., Hoboken: John Wiley & Sons Ltd, 2013, http://books.google.com.

[23] Public Law 110-85 (September 27, 2007).

[24] Institute of Medicine. (2010). Rare Diseases and Orphan Products: Accelerating Research and Development.

[25] Summaries of expedited programs are adapted from: Pariser AR, Robb M, Sherman RE. Expedited programs for drug development and approval. Expert Opinion on Orphan Drugs. 2013;1:507-510.

[26] Priority review is a concept that was created administratively by FDA and that is recognized in the goal letter described in section 101(b) of the Prescription Drug User Fee Amendments of 2012 and in section 529(a)(1) of the FD&C Act.

[27] In addition to these eligibility criteria, there are some types of drugs or drug development programs that have been mandated to receive Fast Track and/or Priority Review status by statute, e.g., qualified infectious disease products under Title VIII of FDASIA entitled "Generating Antibiotic Incentives Now"

[28] Accelerated approval is codified in 21 CFR part 314, subpart H, 21 CFR part 601, subpart E, and referenced in section 506(c) of the FD&C Act, as amended by section 901 of FDASIA.

[29] Fast track is formalized in section 506(b) of the FD&C Act, as added by section 112 of FDAMA and amended by section 901 of FDASIA.

[30] In addition to these eligibility criteria, there are some types of drugs or drug development programs that have been mandated to receive Fast Track and/or Priority Review status by statute, e.g., qualified infectious disease products under Title VIII of FDASIA entitled "Generating Antibiotic Incentives Now"

[31] Break through designation is formalized in section 506(a) of the FD&C Act, as added by section 902 of FDASIA.

[32] Section 513(f)(2) of the FD&C Act was amended by section 607 of FDASIA, on July 9, 2012, to allow a sponsor to submit a de novo classification request to the FDA for novel low to moderate risk devices without first being required to submit a 510(k).

[33] Some examples of recent approvals in 2013 and 2014 include mipomersen for the treatment of homozygous familial hypercholesterolemia; Japanese encephalitis virus vaccine for Japanese encephalitis; elosulfase alfa for the treatment of mucopolysaccharidosis type IVA (Morquio A syndrome); miltefosine for the treatment of leishmaniasis; and coagulation factor IX (recombinant), Fc fusion protein for adults and children with hemophilia B.

[34] Sasinowski, FJ. Quantum of Effectiveness Evidence in FDA's Approval of Orphan Drugs: Cataloguing FDA's Flexibility in Regulating Therapies for Persons with Rare Disorders. Drug Information Journal 2012; 46:238-263. The NORD report presented examples of FDA's flexibility, that historically, FDA has demonstrated flexibility in its review of effectiveness data in two of every three orphan drugs approved.

[35] A Written Request, issued under BPCA, is a specific document from FDA that is signed by the applicable office director(s) in which the Agency requests submission of certain studies to determine if the use of a drug could have meaningful health benefits in the pediatric population. FDA may issue a Written Request for those studies at the request of an interested party or on its own initiative. Issuance of a Written Request to a sponsor does not require the sponsor to conduct pediatric studies described in the Written Request. It is the sponsor's decision whether to conduct the studies and possibly gain pediatric exclusivity.

[36] To be tax-exempt under section 501(c)(3) of the Internal Revenue Code, an organization must be organized and operated exclusively for exempt purposes set forth in section 501(c)(3), and none of its earnings may inure to any private shareholder or individual. In addition, it may not be an *action organization, i.e.,* it may not attempt to influence legislation as a substantial part of its activities and it may not participate in any campaign activity for or against political candidates.

[37] Workgroup members who planned and organized the workshops included representatives from the Center for Drug Evaluation and Research, the Center for Biologics Evaluation and Research, the Center for Devices and Radiological Health, the Office of Orphan Products Development, and the Office of Pediatric Therapeutics.

[38] 21 CFR 814.20(b)(13); 79 Federal Register 7 (10 January 2014), pp. 1735-1741.

[39] The tools, standards, and approaches needed to develop a new medical device, to test that the device is performing as predicted, and to regulate the device for safety and effectiveness.

[40] Institute of Medicine. (2010). Rare Diseases and Orphan Products: Accelerating Research and Development.

[41] Haihao S., et al. Steps Toward Harmonization for Clinical Development of Medicines in Pediatric Ulcerative Colitis—A Global Scientific Discussion, Part 1: Efficacy Endpoints and

Disease Outcome Assessments. Journal of Pediatric Gastroenterology & Nutrition 2014; 58(6):679-683.

[42] Haihao S., et al. Steps Toward Harmonization for Clinical Development of Medicines in Pediatric Ulcerative Colitis—A Global Scientific Discussion, Part 2: Data Extrapolation, Trial Design, and Pharmacokinetics. Journal of Pediatric Gastroenterology & Nutrition 2014; 58(6):684-683.

[43] Biomarkers Definitions Working Group (2001). *Clinical Pharmacology and Therapeutics, 69,* p. 89–95.

[44] Animal models are a third category of DDTs available for qualification. The Animal Model Qualification program is a voluntary program and applies specifically to animal models intended for use in the adequate and well-controlled efficacy studies that serve as substantial evidence of effectiveness for drugs developed under the Animal Rule (See 21 CFR 314.600 for drugs; 21 CFR 601.90 for biological products). Further information on the program can be found on FDA's website "Animal Model Qualification Program".

[45] The term "context of use" refers to a comprehensive description that fully and clearly delineates the limits of FDA's qualification decision in terms of the manner and purpose of use for the DDT(s). The context of use statement should describe all criteria under which the DDT is qualified for use. The qualified context of use defines the boundaries within which the available data adequately justify use of the DDT(s). As data from additional studies are obtained over time, submitters of DDTs may continue working within the DDT Qualification Programs to submit additional data and expand the qualified context of use.

[46] For these purposes, an unmet medical need for devices is a condition, the treatment or diagnosis of which is not addressed adequately by an available therapy or diagnostic, such as, no approved alternative treatment or means of diagnosis exists; or the device offers breakthrough or significant, clinically meaningful advantages over existing approved alternative treatments; or the availability of the device is in the best interest of patients.

[47] See section 515(d) of FD&C Act.

[48] With regard to EAP Devices an "intermediate endpoint" is used in a clinical study as a measurement of clinical benefit or risk concerning a symptom or measure of function that is not the ultimate outcome of the disease, and a "surrogate endpoint" is not itself a measure of clinical benefit, but is used in trials as a substitute which is reasonably likely to predict clinical benefit, based on epidemiologic, therapeutic, pathophysiologic or other scientific evidence.

[49] Although priority review for devices is already established and was created to help expedite patient access to certain devices important to public health, FDA's experience is that review times can take longer for these devices than for other devices reviewed under a PMA because of the novel scientific issues these devices may raise. It is believed that the EAP program may enable patients to have more timely access to these devices because of the earlier involvement of FDA during the device development process.

[50] http://www.fda.gov/drugs/developmentapprovalprocess/howdrugsaredevelopedand approved/ approvalapplications/investig ationalnewdrugindapplication/ucm343349.htm.

[51] http://www.fda.gov/ForIndustry/DevelopingProductsforRareDiseasesConditions/ucm 385535. htm.

In: Drug Development   ISBN: 978-1-53610-227-7
Editor: Frederick Johnston   © 2016 Nova Science Publishers, Inc.

Chapter 2

RARE DISEASES: TOO EARLY TO GAUGE EFFECTIVENESS OF FDA'S PEDIATRIC VOUCHER PROGRAM*

United States Government Accountability Office

ABBREVIATIONS

FDA	Food and Drug Administration
FDASIA	Food and Drug Administration Safety and Innovation Act
HHS	Department of Health and Human Services
NIH	National Institutes of Health

WHY GAO DID THIS STUDY

Almost 7,000 rare diseases, most of which are serious or life-threatening, affect more than 25 million Americans. About half of all rare diseases affect children, and few of these diseases have viable treatments. To encourage the development of drugs to treat or prevent rare pediatric diseases, the Food and Drug Administration Safety and Innovation Act (FDASIA) of 2012 authorized FDA to award a priority review voucher to a drug sponsor upon approval of that

---

* This is an edited, reformatted and augmented version of The United States Government Accountability Office publication, GAO-16-319, dated March 2016.

sponsor's drug to treat a rare pediatric disease. A drug sponsor can later redeem the voucher when submitting another new drug application to treat any disease or condition in adults or children, or sell or transfer the voucher to another sponsor. A voucher entitles a sponsor to a 6-month priority review by FDA rather than the 10-month standard review.

FDASIA included a provision for GAO to study the pediatric voucher program. GAO examined what is known about the effectiveness of the program in encouraging the development of drugs to prevent or treat certain rare pediatric diseases. GAO reviewed relevant laws and documentation related to the program and its management, and identified drug sponsors who were awarded vouchers, the diseases their drugs were approved to treat, and whether the vouchers were redeemed, sold, or transferred. GAO also interviewed FDA officials, drug sponsors, patient advocacy groups, and organizations representing physicians and children's hospitals, among others.

WHAT GAO FOUND

It is too early to gauge whether the Food and Drug Administration's (FDA) pediatric voucher program has stimulated the development of drugs to treat or prevent rare pediatric diseases. Given that the typical drug development process often exceeds a decade, insufficient time has elapsed to determine whether the 3 year-old program has been effective. Any drug sponsors motivated by the program to attempt to develop a drug for a rare pediatric disease may be many years from submitting new drug applications—which contain scientific and clinical data about safety and effectiveness—to FDA for review.

As of December 31, 2015, there have been 11 requests for a pediatric voucher. Of these, six have been awarded, two denied, and three remain under review. The six drugs for which vouchers were awarded were in development prior to the program's implementation and these drugs helped fulfill unmet medical needs. One drug is indicated to treat a rare pediatric cancer, and the other five drugs treat rare metabolic diseases affecting children. No other drugs had been previously approved by FDA for these conditions. Four of the six awarded pediatric vouchers have been sold to other drug sponsors for prices ranging from $67.5 million to $350 million. One of the six vouchers awarded has been redeemed and was used to obtain a priority review of a new drug application for a drug to treat adults with high cholesterol. FDA approved this new drug application in July 2015.

FDA officials stated that, while they strongly support the goal of incentivizing drug development for rare pediatric diseases, they have seen no evidence that the program is effective. The program's authorization, as amended, is set to terminate October 1, 2016, and FDA officials said they do not support the program's continuation. They expressed concern that the program adversely affects the agency's ability to set its public health priorities by requiring FDA to provide priority reviews of new drug applications that would not otherwise qualify if they do not treat a serious condition or provide a significant improvement in safety or effectiveness. Additionally, FDA officials said that the additional workload from the program strains the agency's resources. However, other stakeholders provided generally positive feedback on the program. For example, drug sponsors that sold these vouchers said they plan to reinvest portions of the proceeds they received into additional research on rare pediatric diseases, although there is no requirement to do so. Patient advocacy groups told GAO that the program could lead to the development of needed drugs.

We provided a draft of this report for comment to the Department of Health and Human Services (HHS). HHS provided technical comments, which we incorporated as appropriate.

* * *

March 2, 2016

The Honorable Lamar Alexander
Chairman

The Honorable Patty Murray
Ranking Member
Committee on Health, Education, Labor, and Pensions
United States Senate

The Honorable Fred Upton
Chairman

The Honorable Frank Pallone, Jr.
Ranking Member

Committee on Energy and Commerce
House of Representatives

Rare diseases are diseases that affect fewer than 200,000 people in the United States. However, they pose a serious health concern as approximately 7,000 rare diseases affect more than 25 million Americans, according to the National Institutes of Health (NIH).[1] Almost half of these diseases affect children. The onset of a rare disease can be devastating for patients and their families. Most of these diseases are serious, disabling, and life-threatening, yet little may be known about them, making it difficult to diagnose a patient correctly. Even once a patient is diagnosed, many rare diseases do not have viable treatment options. Individuals with a rare disease can experience shortened life expectancy or decreased quality of life. Finding effective treatments for these diseases is important but challenging, and developing such treatments specifically for children adds to that challenge.

Over the years, a number of laws have been enacted to improve the availability of drugs for patients with rare diseases and for children, including the Orphan Drug Act, the Pediatric Research Equity Act of 2003, and the Best Pharmaceuticals for Children Act.[2] Most recently, in 2012, the Food and Drug Administration Safety and Innovation Act (FDASIA) authorized a new program to encourage the development of new drugs for rare pediatric diseases.[3] Through this program, the sponsor of a new drug application that is approved by the Food and Drug Administration (FDA) may be eligible to receive a voucher entitling it to later receive a 6-month priority review for another of its new drug applications for a drug to treat any disease or condition in adults or children, rather than the typical 10-month standard review.[4] The voucher may also be transferred or sold to another drug sponsor, who may then redeem it.[5] The potential for additional revenue that comes from marketing a drug approximately 4 months sooner—or the proceeds that may come from selling the voucher to another drug sponsor—could incentivize sponsors to develop drugs that prevent or treat rare pediatric diseases.

FDASIA included a provision that we study the effectiveness of the rare pediatric disease priority review voucher program.[6] This report examines what is known about the effectiveness of the pediatric voucher program in encouraging the development of drugs to prevent or treat certain rare pediatric diseases.

To perform our work, we examined relevant laws, policies, FDA guidance, and other documentation related to the pediatric voucher program and its management, including FDASIA's provisions, FDA's draft guidance for industry on pediatric vouchers, and FDA's report on developing drugs for rare pediatric diseases and its strategic plan for accelerating drug development for them.[7] Additionally, we obtained information from FDA about the number of requests FDA has received for pediatric vouchers and related requests for rare pediatric disease designations, which are usually a precursor to receiving a voucher and which a drug sponsor may request any time during the drug development process. In addition, we reviewed information from FDA related to the new drug applications for which vouchers were awarded. We identified drug sponsors that were awarded these vouchers and the diseases their drugs were approved to treat, as well as the status of the vouchers once awarded—that is, whether they had been sold, transferred, or redeemed. We reviewed the medical literature and information from NIH, patient advocacy groups, and physicians to learn about the rare pediatric diseases for which these drugs had been developed, including how patients with these diseases are currently treated.

We interviewed FDA officials to supplement our understanding of the pediatric voucher program, and FDA and NIH officials to supplement our understanding of the diseases for which vouchers were awarded. We also spoke with 9 of the 10 drug sponsors that were awarded, purchased, or otherwise received or redeemed a voucher.[8] Among other things, we discussed their perspectives on the program, including the extent to which they believed the program acted as an incentive for drug sponsors to encourage the development of drugs for rare pediatric diseases. Additionally, we spoke with six patient advocacy groups associated with the rare pediatric diseases for which a voucher was awarded, and with several organizations representing the pharmaceutical industry, the insurance industry, and other interested organizations and individuals.[9] (See app. I for a complete list of those we interviewed.)

We conducted this performance audit from July 2015 to March 2016 in accordance with generally accepted government auditing standards. Those standards require that we plan and perform the audit to obtain sufficient, appropriate evidence to provide a reasonable basis for our findings based on our audit objectives. We believe that the evidence obtained provides a reasonable basis for our findings and conclusions based on our audit objectives.

BACKGROUND

Rare Pediatric Diseases and Drug Development Challenges

A rare pediatric disease, as defined by statute, is one that primarily affects children 18 years and younger and generally affects fewer than 200,000 individuals in the United States.[10] Some diseases affect less than a handful of children, while others affect many more. In many cases, no FDA-approved therapy exists for the treatment of the disease.

Drug development is inherently challenging, and developing drugs to treat rare pediatric diseases adds layers of complexity. The drug development process in general is time-consuming and costly for drug sponsors. The drug industry estimates that, on average, a sponsor spends over a decade developing a drug at an average cost of $2.6 billion.[11] The industry also reports that the percentage of drugs that enter clinical trials and that are eventually approved by FDA as safe and efficacious is less than 12 percent. Many more drugs will fail and prove to be either unsafe or ineffective at the earlier, preclinical stage. Developing drugs to treat rare pediatric diseases is even more challenging for several reasons. By definition, the number of patients affected by any individual rare disease is small, making it difficult to understand a disease's progression and to design studies for potential new drugs. For example, FDA has pointed out that this challenge is further compounded in drug development for children, as they represent a smaller percentage of the overall population, which makes it difficult to identify and recruit sufficient numbers of patients to include in studies.[12] The agency further notes that conducting these studies is difficult because the manifestation and progression of the same rare disease can vary by patient. There can also be different subtypes of a single disease, which can further reduce the number of patients to study. Further, there are relatively few researchers who are knowledgeable about a particular rare disease, which makes designing studies challenging. In addition, according to drug sponsors, there may be a greater incentive for them to focus on developing drugs for large patient populations that produce higher returns on investment than drugs for smaller patient populations that may generate less revenue. As a result of these challenges and others, drug sponsors may be hesitant to attempt to develop drugs to treat rare pediatric diseases.

FDA and the Pediatric Voucher Program

FDA, an agency within the Department of Health and Human Services (HHS), is responsible for overseeing the safety and efficacy of drugs sold in the United States.[13] This responsibility includes the implementation of the pediatric voucher program, as provided for in FDASIA. FDA may award a drug sponsor a voucher upon approval of that sponsor's new drug application for a rare pediatric disease. Specifically, the drug must be for the prevention or treatment of a rare disease that primarily affects children 18 or under.[14] The application may include the same indication for use in adults with the same rare pediatric disease, but it cannot include a different adult indication. Other criteria must also be met in order to receive a voucher. For example, the drug must not contain an active ingredient that has been previously approved by FDA in another drug application, and the drug must be eligible for priority review.[15] New drug applications that FDA determines not to qualify for a priority review, and which therefore receive a standard review, are ineligible to receive a pediatric priority review voucher.

If a drug meets the eligibility criteria, the drug sponsor should include a request for a pediatric voucher in its new drug application, including supporting documentation demonstrating how the application meets the eligibility criteria for a pediatric voucher. Alternatively, if a drug sponsor does not submit a request for a pediatric voucher, but FDA determines that the sponsor may be eligible to receive one, FDA notifies the drug sponsor of its possible eligibility. Once FDA receives a sponsor's new drug application and pediatric voucher request, it reviews the information and considers whether it should be approved. If FDA approves the drug application, it includes its decision regarding whether to award a pediatric voucher in its approval letter. In making this decision, FDA determines whether the drug sponsor has met all of the eligibility criteria for a pediatric voucher, which includes determining that the drug is for a rare pediatric disease as well as reviewing the clinical data examining the drug's use in a pediatric population included in the drug application.

Once a drug sponsor is awarded a voucher, it can later be redeemed by that sponsor with the submission of another new drug application for a drug to treat any disease or condition in adults or children, making the sponsor automatically eligible for a 6-month priority review. The original drug sponsor also has the option of selling or transferring the voucher to a new drug sponsor, who may then choose to use the voucher or similarly sell or transfer it.[16] The voucher may be transferred any number of times before it is used.[17] When the sponsor who possesses the voucher ultimately decides to redeem it, the sponsor must notify

FDA at least 90 days in advance of submitting the new drug application.[18] The sponsor redeeming the voucher must also pay any other required user fees.[19] Figure 1 provides a general overview of the pediatric voucher program.

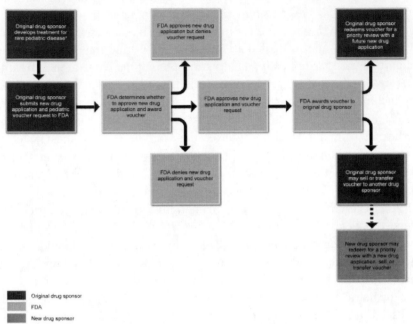

Original drug sponsor

FDA

New drug sponsor

Source: GAO analysis of FDA information. | GAO-16-319.

Note: Among other things, a new drug application submitted by a sponsor seeking a pediatric priority review voucher must itself be deemed eligible by FDA for a priority review. New drug applications that FDA determines not to qualify for a priority review, and which therefore receive a standard review, are ineligible to receive a pediatric priority review voucher.

[a] Prior to submitting a new drug application, a drug sponsor may request a rare pediatric disease designation. To receive such designation, the sponsor must provide information supporting why it concludes that the disease is rare and primarily affects children. FDA encourages drug sponsors to request this designation to ensure, for example, that the agency has the necessary information to later evaluate a drug's pediatric voucher eligibility. In the absence of a sponsor designation request, FDA may request and review supporting documentation from the sponsor in order to verify that a disease qualifies as rare and pediatric.

Figure 1. General Overview of the Rare Pediatric Disease Priority Review Voucher Program, as of December 2015.

Before submitting a new drug application, a sponsor may also request a rare pediatric disease designation for a drug that is still in development. This designation was established as part of the pediatric voucher program in 2012.[20] In its designation request, a sponsor is to include information about, among other things, the drug and the rare pediatric disease for which the drug is being investigated, and the basis for concluding that the disease is rare and primarily affects children. FDA reviews the provided information and generally informs a drug sponsor of its designation decision within 60 days of receiving the request. FDA encourages drug sponsors to request such a designation in order for the agency to have the necessary information to evaluate a drug's pediatric voucher eligibility and to ensure that drug sponsors have an adequate opportunity to provide this information before requesting a voucher. However, requesting such designation is not required in order to receive a rare pediatric disease voucher. If a rare pediatric disease designation is not requested prior to a drug sponsor submitting its new drug application, FDA officials may determine through their reviews of a new drug application and discussions with a drug sponsor that a certain drug may be eligible for a voucher. FDA officials will ask the drug sponsor to submit the necessary information to demonstrate that the drug is for a rare pediatric disease as, according to FDA, that information is generally not included in a new drug application.

TOO EARLY TO GAUGE IF PEDIATRIC VOUCHER PROGRAM STIMULATES DRUG DEVELOPMENT

Drugs for Which Vouchers Were Awarded Were in Development Prior to the Program's Implementation, though They Helped Fulfill Unmet Medical Need

Given that the typical drug development process often exceeds a decade, insufficient time has elapsed to gauge whether the 3-year-old pediatric voucher program has been effective at encouraging the development of drugs for rare pediatric diseases. We found that each of the drugs awarded pediatric vouchers were in development prior to the voucher program's implementation. Any sponsors motivated by this relatively new program to attempt to develop drugs for such diseases would likely be years away from submitting their new drug applications to FDA.

Although it is too early to gauge whether the program stimulates drug development, a potential indication of sponsor interest in the program may be reflected by the number of requests that have been submitted for a pediatric voucher or a rare pediatric disease designation. We examined how many requests for pediatric vouchers and rare pediatric disease designation were submitted to FDA and how many of these vouchers were awarded and designations were granted. As of December 31, 2015, there have been 11 requests for a pediatric voucher. Of these, 6 have been awarded, 2 denied, and 3 are still under review.[21] The fact that the sponsors of these drugs took the steps to request vouchers and demonstrate their eligibility—either on their own initiative or in response to FDA's suggestion—suggests interest in the program. Similarly, taking steps to demonstrate that their drugs are intended to treat rare pediatric diseases and requesting such designations also indicates that these sponsors are considering applying for a pediatric voucher. Since the pediatric voucher program and designation were established, through December 31, 2015, there have been 52 rare pediatric disease designations requested and 29 granted.[22] Because requests for a rare pediatric disease designation can be submitted at any time in the drug development process prior to submitting a new drug application, these designations could be for drugs that, for example, are in early stages of development and were pursued specifically in response to the program. Alternatively, these designations could be for drugs that were being studied before FDASIA was enacted and thus are farther along in the development process. According to FDA, the agency does not track which stage of development a drug is in when a request for this designation is submitted.

The six drugs for which pediatric vouchers were awarded helped fulfill an unmet medical need. Specifically, these six drugs were the first drugs approved by FDA to treat the seven rare pediatric diseases for which they are indicated. No other drugs had been previously approved for these diseases.

- Vimizim, sponsored by BioMarin Pharmaceutical, treats children with Mucopolysaccharidosis Type IVA, a rare inherited metabolic disorder resulting from an enzyme deficiency. According to FDA and NIH, the drug significantly improves patients' ability to walk.
- Unituxin, sponsored by United Therapeutics, is intended to help patients with high-risk neuroblastoma, a rare pediatric cancer, and, according to FDA, improves the overall survival rates of affected children.
- Cholbam, sponsored by Asklepion Pharmaceuticals, is considered by relevant patient advocacy groups to be an effective and important

therapy for children with some bile acid synthesis disorders and some peroxisomal disorders, both of which are metabolic disorders.

- Xuriden, sponsored by Wellstat Therapeutics, allows certain children with hereditary orotic aciduria—an extremely rare, genetic metabolic disorder—to live life unimpeded by the disease as long as they continue treatment, according to FDA.

- Strensiq, sponsored by Alexion Pharmaceuticals, is for use by children suffering from hypophosphatasia, a genetic, rare metabolic disorder. FDA and physicians reported that the drug increased survival rates and alleviated symptoms among children in clinical trials

- Kanuma, also sponsored by Alexion Pharmaceuticals, is for use by patients with lysosomal acid lipase deficiency, a rare, genetic, progressive metabolic disorder. According to FDA, the drug demonstrated increased life expectancy in a clinical trial among children who were diagnosed as infants.

Officials from both NIH and FDA agree that these drugs are meaningful for patients with the rare pediatric diseases as the drugs may, for example, increase life expectancy, alleviate certain symptoms, or otherwise improve quality of life. Similarly, patient advocacy groups and physicians said that these drugs provide important new treatment for patients and improve survival rates and symptoms. (See app. II for a summary about each of these diseases based on information available from NIH, patient advocacy groups, and physicians familiar with these diseases.)

As of December 31, 2015, four of the six pediatric vouchers—for Vimizim, Unituxin, Cholbam, and Xuriden—have been sold or transferred to other drug sponsors. Sale prices of the pediatric vouchers have ranged from $67.5 million to $350 million.[23] The other two awarded vouchers—for Strensiq and Kanuma—remain held by the original sponsor. Only the voucher awarded for Vimizim has been redeemed. It was used to expedite the review of Praluent, a new drug to treat adults with high cholesterol. See table 1 for more detailed information about the status of these vouchers.

Table 1. Status of the Rare Pediatric Disease Priority Review Vouchers Awarded to Drug Sponsors by FDA as of December 31, 2015

Drug	Date voucher awarded and drug sponsor	Status of voucher	Sale price of voucher	Details on voucher redemption
Vimizim (elosulfase alfa), to treat Mucopolysaccharidosis Type IVA (Morquio A syndrome)	February 14, 2014; BioMarin Pharmaceutical	Sold to Regeneron Pharmaceuticals; transferred to Sanofi[a]	$67.5 million	Redeemed November 24, 2014, for Praluent (anew cholesterol drug) approved by FDA July 24, 2015[b]
Unituxin (dinutuximab), to treat patients with high-risk neuroblastoma	March 10, 2015; United Therapeutics	Sold to AbbVie	$350 million	N/A
Cholbam (cholic acid), to treat (1) bile acid synthesis disorders due to single enzyme defects, and (2) peroxisomal disorders (including Zellweger spectrum disorders)	March 17, 2015; Asklepion Pharmaceuticals	Transferred to Retrophin as part of a purchasing agreement;[c] later sold to Sanofi	Unable to quantify price of first transfer; then sold for $245 million	N/A
Xuriden (uridine triacetate), to treat hereditary orotic aciduria	September 4, 2015; Wellstat Therapeutics	Sold to AstraZeneca	Financial terms of the voucher sale are unavailable	N/A
Strensiq (asfotase alfa), to treat hypophosphatasia	October 23, 2015; Alexion Pharmaceuticals	Unsold	N/A	N/A
Kanuma (sebelipase alfa), to treat lysosomal acid lipase deficiency	December 8, 2015; Alexion Pharmaceuticals	Unsold	N/A	N/A

Source: GAO summary of FDA and drug sponsor information. | GAO-16-319.

[a] Regeneron purchased the voucher from BioMarin. Regeneron and another drug sponsor, Sanofi, collaborated to develop Praluent. According to these two drug

sponsors, they shared the purchase price of the voucher equally. Regeneron transferred the voucher to Sanofi, who redeemed it with FDA for Praluent.

b Under the most recent reauthorization of the Prescription Drug User Fee Act in 2012, one of FDA's goals is to complete a priority review of a new drug application within 6 months and a standard review within 10 months of the 60-day filing date. This means a priority review can take up to 8 months, and a standard review up to 12 months. Operating under this goal, FDA achieved its goal of a priority review for Praluent.

c Retrophin purchased Cholbam and related assets, including the voucher, from Asklepion. As a result, the voucher was transferred from Asklepion to Retrophin under the terms of the agreement.

FDA Does Not Believe the Pediatric Voucher Program Effectively Stimulates Drug Development and Opposes Its Reauthorization

FDA officials expressed concern about the pediatric voucher program, and do not support its continuation after its current authorization expires October 1, 2016. In written responses to our questions, FDA officials reported that they have seen no evidence that the program has encouraged increased development of drugs for rare pediatric diseases. The agency also indicated that while it strongly supports the goal of the program—incentivizing the development of drugs for rare pediatric diseases—it has not seen evidence that the program has yet been effective in achieving this goal. Instead, the agency suggested that companies may consider that other incentives, such as provision of an additional period of "market exclusivity," may be more effective at incentivizing drug development than the priority review vouchers.[24] FDA specifically cited its authority to provide an additional 6 months of market exclusivity for FDA requested pediatric studies in products that may produce health benefits in the pediatric population—known as pediatric exclusivity—as providing an effective incentive to drug sponsors.[25]

In addition to sharing its views regarding the program's effectiveness in incentivizing drug development, FDA cited concerns about what it considers to be the significant adverse impact of the program on the agency's ability to determine its public health priorities. According to FDA, the program interferes with its ability to set priorities on the basis of public health needs by requiring FDA to provide priority reviews of new drug applications that would not otherwise qualify, based on the merits of those applications. The agency noted that an application for a drug will receive priority review designation if it is for a drug that treats a serious condition and, if approved, would provide a significant improvement in safety or effectiveness. However, FDA anticipates that sponsors will seek to redeem their vouchers for new drug applications that would otherwise receive a standard 10-month review for more prevalent conditions that already have available treatments. Such applications may be for drugs to treat diseases or conditions such as elevated blood pressure, high cholesterol, obesity, or diabetes and other drugs with substantial market potential. FDA explained that, in effect, the program allows sponsors to "purchase" a priority review at the expense of other important public health work in FDA's portfolio, which undermines FDA's public health mission and the morale of its professional review staff.

According to FDA, the pediatric voucher program also places a substantial strain on its workload. First, the agency explained that performing a priority review on a drug that would otherwise merit a standard review requires the agency to conduct significant work in a compressed timeframe. FDA pointed out that, while patients and providers are willing to accept a greater risk for a drug that fulfills an unmet medical need, there is a different benefit risk balance that must be considered when assessing drugs for more prevalent conditions that may be used in millions of patients. A new drug application qualifying for a standard review is typically accompanied by very large data sets, reflective of the study of thousands of patients to support substantial evidence of the drug's effectiveness and to provide the safety data required to demonstrate that its benefits outweigh its risks. As a result, 6- month priority reviews of applications that would otherwise receive a 10- month standard review require FDA to conduct work in 4 months less time. FDA noted that, in order to meet the required shortened timeframe for review, staff must divert attention from other important work or management must assign more reviewers to review an application. FDA noted that it confronted this challenge and had to curtail or defer other important work with the first redemption of a pediatric voucher for Praluent.

Second, FDA indicated that the pediatric voucher program hinders its ability to effectively manage its own workload. FDA pointed out that it is organized into separate review divisions with specific areas of expertise and that it cannot quickly train new staff. There is not a pool of review staff that can be moved from one review division to another review division on an ad hoc basis to complete priority reviews for the application based on the rare pediatric review vouchers. According to FDA, it cannot predict which review divisions will need additional staff to complete the additional priority reviews, making anticipatory hiring infeasible. Although FDA receives a special user fee from a drug sponsor when the sponsor redeems a voucher, in addition to the regular user fee that accompanies a new drug application, the agency noted that FDASIA did not authorize resources beyond the user fees—funding or staff—to administer the program, including determining rare pediatric disease designations. FDA noted that there is a disconnect in the timing of its collection of the additional user fee and the time it takes the agency to hire, orient, and train additional reviewers to assist with the additional reviews. Furthermore, the additional user fee is a one-time payment and does not provide the funding needed to sustain the longer-term employment of additional staff hired to assist with conducting the priority review. While the additional user fee is intended to compensate for FDA's increased workload related to redemption of the vouchers, FDA noted that the funding mechanism does not provide the agency the resources required to review the particular voucher priority application. FDA told us that, if the number of pediatric vouchers awarded and redeemed continues to increase, the agency's ability to meet its public health mission and other commitments will be adversely affected, including monitoring postmarket safety, engaging with patient and stakeholder groups, and advising drug sponsors on their development programs, including those focused on pediatric drugs.

Third, in a discussion with FDA, officials said that the pediatric voucher program has also significantly increased its workload due to its need to respond to requests for rare pediatric disease designations, often within 60 days, and the complexity involved in making such determinations.[26] Determining whether to designate a drug as one for a rare pediatric disease is challenging; FDA officials told us that the vast majority of initial requests for such designation have not included adequate information to demonstrate that the disease primarily affects children 18 years and younger. As a result, FDA must work with the drug sponsor to determine what types of information are acceptable to support such an assertion.

Drug Sponsors, Advocacy Groups, and Other Organizations Generally Support the Pediatric Voucher Program

Feedback from stakeholders about the pediatric voucher program varied but has been generally positive, with nearly all drug sponsors and patient advocacy groups we spoke with saying that the program could potentially motivate further research in rare pediatric diseases. Drug sponsors largely favor the program; one sponsor and half of the patient advocacy groups with whom we spoke pointed to the sales of and prices for the vouchers as evidence that demand for the vouchers exists. Most sponsors also noted that each sale provides cash infusions for drug sponsors who were initially awarded—and later sold—the vouchers. Four of five sponsors that were awarded or transferred and later sold vouchers told us that they plan to reinvest a portion of the proceeds they received into additional research and development of drugs to treat other rare pediatric diseases. However, there is no requirement that sponsors must use the proceeds in this way. A few sponsors said that the program will be a factor in future business decisions and most said that it will likely encourage the development of drugs for treating rare pediatric diseases if it is reauthorized.

Patient advocacy groups also generally favor the program. For example, one group we spoke to said that the program has stimulated a transfer of cash from larger drug sponsors to smaller ones through the sales of the vouchers, and that these smaller drug sponsors may reinvest a portion of the proceeds to continue developing drugs for rare pediatric diseases. A few groups also indicated that the program could lead to the development of much-needed pediatric drugs without costing the government resources.[27] Most told us that they believe the program incentivizes drug development. A few groups told us that, since the creation of the program, they have spoken with several drug sponsors interested in discussing the extent to which their drugs in development might be able to treat the patients that these groups represent.

Although sponsors and patient advocacy groups were generally positive about the voucher program, some also expressed concerns related to the uncertain future of the program and FDA's interpretation of what diseases are considered rare pediatric diseases, concerns also expressed by organizations representing physicians and the health insurance industry. For example, some of the sponsors, patient advocacy groups, and other organizations that we contacted said that the FDASIA provision providing for termination of FDA's authority to award pediatric vouchers one year after the award of the third voucher under the program (March 2016) created ambiguity for industry that therefore diminishes the program's appeal.[28] Specifically, two drug sponsors told us that they are concerned about pursuing lengthy and costly drug development for rare pediatric diseases in order to obtain a voucher that may be unavailable by the time they are ready to submit new drug applications to FDA. To enhance the program's effectiveness, most drug sponsors and many patient advocacy groups said that they believe the program should be reauthorized for a longer period of time, or even permanently. Additionally, a drug sponsor and a few patient advocacy groups told us that, in their view, FDA's interpretation of the definition of a rare pediatric disease is too narrow. Some said that as a result, certain rare diseases, such as sickle cell disease and some pediatric cancers, are not eligible for a pediatric voucher because more than 50 percent of afflicted children survive to adulthood.[29] One patient advocacy group indicated that such an exclusion effectively penalizes all patients with these diseases because a majority of them live past 18 years, although the onset of the disease occurs during childhood. They told us that they believe such diseases should be included in FDA's definition. When asked about how the agency determined its definition of a rare pediatric disease, FDA officials pointed out that a vast majority of rare diseases are diagnosed in childhood— given this, products for all rare diseases diagnosed at that time would be eligible for a voucher. However, since children were to be the intended population for pediatric voucher program per FDASIA, FDA officials noted that, by law, the definition applies to those diseases that primarily affect children 18 years and younger.

Several drug sponsors and a patient advocacy group raised some concerns about the program but were uncertain about how to address them. For example, certain drug sponsors and the patient advocacy group suggested that there might be an optimal number of vouchers to be awarded to maximize their value to industry and their incentivizing effect. The patient advocacy group suggested that awarding too many vouchers would cause their value to plummet. However, most of them were uncertain about what the optimum quantity of awarded vouchers should be. In addition, similar to a concern raised by FDA, one drug sponsor told us that it was concerned that incentivizing development of drugs for rare pediatric diseases could potentially lead to unintended consequences, such as diverting attention from mass-market diseases such as diabetes.

Finally, feedback from organizations representing physicians, health insurers, and children's hospitals about the pediatric voucher program was varied. While two of these organizations generally favored the program, all told us that there was insufficient information to judge the program's overall effectiveness or that it was simply too soon to tell. One organization shared FDA's concerns about potential unintended consequences, such as the diversion of resources from other agency priorities. Feedback from the academic community was also varied. One academic told us that the voucher program has been consistent with his expectations and echoed what a few patient advocacy groups said—that the program could be a stimulant for developing drugs for rare pediatric diseases at little cost to the federal government. In contrast, another academic said it was difficult to determine whether the program stimulated research since only a few years have elapsed since the program was implemented. He indicated, similar to FDA's concern, that the program could instead lead to unintended consequences. For example, this academic suggested that the program could strain FDA resources, commoditize its approval process, and result in the granting of a priority review to a drug that is neither novel nor fulfills an unmet medical need. He also proposed that, if the pediatric voucher program is reauthorized it could be improved by delaying the awarding of the vouchers until several years after the drugs' approval. This would allow more time to assess whether patients have actually benefitted from the drugs, and are able to access the drugs, before the voucher is awarded.

AGENCY COMMENTS

We provided a draft of this report for comment to HHS. HHS provided technical comments, which we incorporated as appropriate.

Marcia Crosse
Director, Health Care

APPENDIX I: LIST OF ORGANIZATIONS AND INDIVIDUALS INTERVIEWED

Federal agencies	1.Department of Health and Human Services, Food and DrugAdministration
	2.Department of Health and Human Services, National Institutes of Health
Drug sponsors	1.Alexion Pharmaceuticals Inc.
	2.Asklepion Pharmaceuticals LLC
	3.AstraZeneca Pharmaceuticals LP
	4.BioMarin Pharmaceutical Inc.
	5.Regeneron Pharmaceuticals, Inc.
	6.Retrophin, Inc.
	7.Sanofi
	8.United Therapeutics Corporation
	9.Wellstat Therapeutics Corporation
Drug sponsor associations	1. Pharmaceutical Research and Manufacturers of America
	2.Biotechnology Industry Organization
Patient advocacy groups	1.National Organization for Rare Disorders
	2.EveryLife Foundation for Rare Diseases

3.Kids v Cancer

4.Children's Neuroblastoma Cancer Foundation

5.Global Foundation for Peroxisomal Disorders

6.Council for Bile Acid Deficiency Diseases

7.National MPS [mucopolysaccharidoses] Society

8.Sickle Cell Disease Association of America, Inc.

9.Soft Bones

10.LAL [lysosomal acid lipase] Solace

Other organizations or individuals

1.American Academy of Pediatrics

2.Children's Hospital Association

3.America's Health Insurance Plans

4.Jerry Vockley, MD., Ph.D.

Professor of Pediatrics and Human Genetics

University of Pittsburgh

5.Dr. David Ridley

Duke University

The Fuqua School of Business

Faculty Director of the Health Sector Management Program

6. Aaron S. Kesselheim, M.D., J.D., M.P.H.

Associate Professor of Medicine, Harvard Medical School Director, Program On Regulation, Therapeutics, And Law Division of Pharmacoepidemiology and Pharmacoeconomics Brigham and Women's Hospital

APPENDIX II: INFORMATION ABOUT THE RARE PEDIATRIC DISEASES THAT CAN BE TREATED BY VOUCHERS WE AWARDED NEWLY APPROVED DRUGS FOR WHICH PEDIATRIC VOUCHERS WERE AWARDED

Pediatric patients affected by seven diseases that previously had no approved treatment may now benefit from six newly-approved drugs for which pediatric vouchers were awarded. We have summarized information about each of these diseases obtained from the National Institutes of Health's Genetics Home Reference, patient advocacy groups, and physicians familiar with these conditions.[1]

MUCOPOLYSACCHARIDOSIS TYPE IVA

Mucopolysaccharidosis type IVA, also known as Morquio A Syndrome, is a rare, progressive, hereditary disease that mainly affects the skeleton and can lead to paralysis and early death. Genetic mutations reduce or eliminate the activity of certain enzymes that are involved in the breakdown of large sugar molecules, resulting in the accumulation of such molecules to toxic levels in many tissues and organs, particularly in the bones, causing deformities. Affected individuals typically demonstrate signs of the disease during early childhood, including skeletal abnormalities such as knock knees, short stature, and abnormalities of the chest, hips, ribs, spine, and wrists. Other symptoms may include vision loss; hearing loss; frequent upper respiratory infections; thin tooth enamel and multiple cavities; heart valve abnormalities; and a mildly-enlarged liver. Morquio A Syndrome does not affect intelligence.

Although the exact prevalence of Morquio A Syndrome is unknown, it is estimated that the broader condition—Mucopolysaccharidosis type IV— occurs in approximately 1 in every 200,000 to 300,000 individuals. The life expectancy of individuals with Morquio A Syndrome depends on the severity of symptoms, with the most severely affected patients surviving only until late childhood or adolescence. Individuals with milder forms of the disorder may live into adulthood, although their life expectancy may be reduced.

Vimizim (elosulfase alfa), is the first FDA-approved drug for the treatment of Morquio A Syndrome. No other FDA-approved therapies exist for treatment of this disease.

HIGH-RISK NEUROBLASTOMA

Neuroblastoma, a type of pediatric cancer that occurs when immature nerve cells become abnormal and multiply uncontrollably, most often occurs in children before age 5 and rarely occurs in adults. Most commonly, a tumor forms in the adrenal gland located above each kidney and can spread to other parts of the body such as the bones, liver, or skin. Tumors also commonly grow in the nerve tissue in the abdomen, chest, neck, or pelvis. Individuals with neuroblastoma may exhibit symptoms such as fever, irritability, pain, tiredness, diarrhea, loss of appetite, and weight loss. Some symptoms may be location-specific, such as a tumor in the abdomen causing abdominal swelling; a tumor in the chest causing difficulty breathing; and a tumor metastasizing to the bone causing bone pain, bruises, and pale skin.

Neuroblastoma occurs in approximately 1 in every 100,000 children and is diagnosed in about 650 children each year in the United States. It is the most common cancer in infants younger than 1 year. Only 40 to 50 percent of children with high-risk neuroblastoma live at least 5 years after diagnosis.

Unituxin (dinutuximab) is the first FDA-approved drug for the treatment of high-risk neuroblastoma. There are currently other FDA-approved drugs for neuroblastoma (specifically, Cyclophosphamide, Vincasar PFS, and Doxorubicin Hydrochloride); however, none of these were approved specifically for the treatment of patients with high-risk neuroblastoma.

BILE ACID SYNTHESIS DISORDERS

Bile acid synthesis disorders are a group of rare metabolic disorders characterized by impaired production and release of a digestive fluid, called bile, from liver cells. People with bile acid synthesis disorders cannot produce bile acids, which are a component of bile that stimulate bile flow and help it absorb fats and fat-soluble vitamins, such as vitamins A, D, E, and K. Consequently, an abnormal form of bile is produced. The failure to produce normal or functional bile acids results in the accumulation of abnormal bile acids and other substances that normally would be broken down within the body, leading to deterioration of certain organ systems. Symptoms may include interruption or suppression of the flow of bile from the liver, fat-soluble vitamin malabsorption, progressive neurological disease, and liver disease.

Bile acid synthesis disorders are estimated to occur in between 1 to 9 individuals in every 1,000,000 births. If left untreated, the disorders may lead to cirrhosis of the liver and death in childhood.

Cholbam (cholic acid) is the first FDA-approved drug for the treatment of bile acid synthesis disorders due to single enzyme defects. No other FDA-approved therapies exist for these disorders.

PEROXISOMAL DISORDERS

Peroxisomal disorders are a group of metabolic disorders, including those in the Zellweger spectrum. These systemic diseases, which affect multiple organs and may have neurological manifestations, present as rare autosomal recessive disorders with impairment of production and release of digestive fluid, called bile, from liver cells. Bile is used during digestion to absorb fats and fat-soluble vitamins, such as vitamins A, D, E, and K. Individuals with the most severe forms of this disease develop symptoms of the condition as newborns, and experience weak muscle tone, feeding problems, hearing and vision loss, and seizures. They may also develop life-threatening problems in other organs and tissues, such as the liver, heart, and kidneys, and may have skeletal abnormalities. Affected individuals have distinctive facial features, including a flattened face and broad nasal bridge. Individuals with less-severe forms of the disease may not develop signs of the disease until late infancy or early childhood. They may have many of the same features as those patients with severe cases; however, their conditions typically progress more slowly. Children with these less-severe conditions often exhibit developmental delays and intellectual disability.

Zellweger spectrum disorders (a subset of peroxisomal disorders) are estimated to occur in approximately 1 in every 50,000 individuals. Peroxisomal disorders encompass a spectrum of disorders, which means the life expectancy of a patient depends on the severity of his or her disease. Patients diagnosed with the most severe form typically do not live beyond 1 year. Children with less severe forms generally live until 10 years of age, although there have been cases reported of children living longer.

Cholbam (cholic acid) is the first FDA-approved drug for the treatment of peroxisomal disorders (including Zellweger spectrum disorders). No other FDA-approved therapies exist for these disorders.

HEREDITARY OROTIC ACIDURIA

Hereditary orotic aciduria is an extremely rare, potentially life-threatening, genetic disorder in which patients cannot produce adequate amounts of uridine, a component of ribonucleic acid that is involved in the synthesis of protein in the body. Patients with inadequate amount of uridine can suffer from blood abnormalities, failure to thrive, a range of developmental delays, and episodes of crystal formation in the urine leading to obstruction of the ureter (a tube that carries urine from the kidneys to the bladder), causing urine to back up into the kidney, making it swell.

Hereditary orotic aciduria is extremely rare, with only four known patients with this disease in the United States, and an estimated 20 worldwide. Left untreated, the disease can contribute to early mortality.

Xuriden (uridine triacetate) is the first FDA-approved drug for the treatment of hereditary orotic aciduria. No other FDA-approved therapies exist for this disease.

HYPOPHOSPHATASIA

Hypophosphatasia is a rare, genetic, progressive, metabolic disease in which patients experience devastating effects on multiple systems of the body, leading to severe physical disability and life-threatening complications. With a spectrum of symptoms and severity, the disease is characterized by defective bone mineralization and softening of the bones. Though forms of hypophosphatasia may appear in childhood or adulthood, the most severe forms tend to occur before birth and in early infancy. Affected newborns exhibit short limbs, an abnormally-shaped chest, and soft skull bones. Additional complications in infancy include poor feeding, a failure to gain weight, respiratory problems, and high levels of calcium in the blood that may lead to kidney problems. Early loss of primary (baby) teeth is one of the first signs of the condition in children. Affected children may have short stature with bowed legs or knock knees, enlarged wrist and ankle joints, and an abnormal skull shape. Afflicted individuals may exhibit delayed development with traditional milestones such as sitting, crawling, or walking.

Severe forms of hypophosphatasia are estimated to occur in approximately 1 in every 100,000 births. Milder cases, such as those that appear in childhood or adulthood, may occur more frequently. The life expectancy of a patient depends on which form of hypophosphatasia (perinatal, infantile, juvenile, or adult) he or she has. The life expectancy of those with the most severe form, perinatal hypophosphatasia, is measured only in days or weeks.

Strensiq (asfotase alfa) is the first FDA-approved drug for the treatment of perinatal, infantile, and juvenile-onset hypophosphatasia. No other FDA-approved therapies exist for this disease.

LYSOSOMAL ACID LIPASE DEFICIENCY

Lysosomal acid lipase deficiency is an inherited spectrum condition in which affected individuals are unable to properly breakdown and use fats and cholesterol in the body. The condition ranges from the infantile-onset form (Wolman disease) to later-onset forms (known as cholesteryl ester storage disease). In affected individuals, harmful amounts of fats may accumulate in areas such as the spleen, liver, bone marrow, and small intestine. Chronic liver disease can develop, along with accumulation of fatty deposits in the arteries. The deposits may eventually block the arteries, which may increase the chance of having a heart attack or stroke. The symptoms of lysosomal acid lipase deficiency are highly variable. Individuals in which onset occurs later in life may experience mild symptoms that are undiagnosed until late adulthood, while those with early onset of the disease may have liver dysfunction in early childhood. Infants with Wolman disease may demonstrate an enlarged liver and spleen, poor weight gain, low muscle tone, jaundice, vomiting, diarrhea, developmental delay, anemia, and poor absorption of nutrients from food.

Wolman disease is estimated to occur in 1 in 350,000 newborns. Children affected by Wolman disease develop severe malnutrition and generally do not survive past early childhood. Comparatively, about 50 individuals affected by cholesteryl ester storage disease have been reported worldwide, and the lifespan of these individuals depends on the severity of the associated complications.

Kanuma (sebelipase alfa) is the first FDA-approved drug for the treatment of lysosomal acid lipase deficiency. No other FDA-approved therapies exist for this disease.

End Notes

[1] See National Institutes of Health, "Fact Sheet: Rare Diseases Clinical Research Network," accessed Dec. 15, 2015, http://report.nih.gov/nihfactsheets/Pdfs/RareDiseasesClinical ResearchNetwork%28ORDR %29.pdf.
[2] Pub. L. No. 97-414, 96 Stat. 2049 (1983) (codified as amended at 21 U.S.C. §§ 360aa et seq. and scattered sections of 15, 21, 26 and 42 U.S.C.). Pub. L. No. 108-155, 117 Stat. 1936 (codified as amended at 21 U.S.C. § 355c). Pub. L. No. 107-109, 115 Stat. 1408 (2002) (codified as amended at 21 U.S.C. §355a and scattered sections of 21 and 42 U.S.C.).
[3] Pub. L. No. 112-144, § 908, 126 Stat. 993, 1094 (2012) (codified as amended at 21 U.S.C. § 360ff). FDASIA included a provision providing for termination of FDA's authority to award pediatric vouchers, 1 year after the date that the third voucher was awarded. 21 U.S.C. § 360ff(b)(5). Subsequent legislation specified that this authority terminates, October 1, 2016. See Consolidated Appropriations Act 2016, Pub. L. No. 114-113, § 765, 129 Stat. 2242, 2287.

[4] Typically, a drug may be eligible for priority review if it is for a serious condition and, if approved, would provide significant improvement in safety and effectiveness—the goal is to complete the priority review in 6 months. In this case, a pediatric voucher gives a sponsor the opportunity to obtain a priority review for a new drug application when it would otherwise be reviewed through FDA's standard review process, which takes approximately 10 months. A new drug application contains scientific and clinical data about a drug's safety and effectiveness. A drug sponsor is the person or entity who assumes responsibility for the marketing of a new drug, including responsibility for complying with applicable laws and regulations.

[5] 21 U.S.C. §360ff(b)(2).

[6] For the purposes of this report, we use the term "pediatric voucher program" to refer to the rare pediatric disease priority review voucher program.

[7] See FDA, Rare Pediatric Disease Priority Review Vouchers, Guidance for Industry, Draft Guidance (Silver Spring, Md.: Nov. 17, 2014), and Report: Complex Issues in Developing Drugs and Biological Products for Rare Diseases and Accelerating the Development of Therapies for Pediatric Rare Diseases Including Strategic Plan: Accelerating the Development of Therapies for Pediatric Rare Disease (Silver Spring, Md.: July 2014).

[8] One of the drug sponsors who purchased a pediatric voucher, AbbVie, declined to speak with us.

[9] We were unable to identify a patient advocacy group representing the rare pediatric disease, hereditary orotic aciduria.

[10] See 21 U.S.C. § 360ff(a)(3).

[11] See Pharmaceutical Research and Manufacturers of America, 2015 Biopharmaceutical Research Industry Profile (Washington, D.C.: April 2015).

[12] See FDA Report: Complex Issues in Developing Drugs.

[13] Unless otherwise indicated, we use the term "drug" to refer to both chemically synthesized drugs and therapeutic biological products in this report. Biological products— which include vaccines, blood products, and proteins—are derived from living sources such as humans, animals, and microorganisms, while drugs are chemically synthesized. We use the term "new drug application" to refer to both new drug applications and biologics license applications submitted to FDA for review.

[14] To date, the drugs for which vouchers have been awarded are indicated to treat rare pediatric diseases. No voucher has been awarded for a new drug application to prevent a rare pediatric disease.

[15] Generally, FDA classifies a drug application eligible for priority review if it treats a serious condition and, when compared to the products that are already on the market, the drug would provide relatively significant improvements in safety or effectiveness. Examples of significant improvements include increased effectiveness in the treatment of a disease or evidence of safety and effectiveness in a new subpopulation. Applications for those drugs with little or no additional therapeutic benefits compared to existing products are classified by FDA as standard. FDA's goal is to complete the review of a priority application within 6 months and a standard application within 10 months.

[16] However, FDA may revoke any pediatric voucher if the rare pediatric disease drug for which the pediatric voucher was awarded is not marketed in the United States within 1 year following the date of approval. 21 U.S.C. § 360ff(e)(1).

[17] Each person to whom a voucher is transferred must notify FDA of the change of voucher ownership within 30 days. 21 U.S.C. § 360ff(b)(2)(B).

[18] 21 U.S.C. § 360ff(b)(4)(A).

[19] FDA is authorized to collect user fees to provide additional resources for FDA to support the process of reviewing applications for new drugs. 21 U.S.C. § 379h. Additionally, priority review user fees are collected from drug sponsors redeeming one of two types of priority review vouchers—for a rare pediatric disease or a tropical disease—to cover FDA's additional costs incurred from reviewing drug applications submitted with these vouchers. 21 U.S.C. §§ 360ff(c) 360n(c). For fiscal year 2016, the rare pediatric disease priority review fee is approximately $2.7 million.

[20] 21 U.S.C. § 360ff(d).

[21] Two pediatric voucher requests were denied because the diseases for which the drugs were under development to treat did not satisfy the definition of a rare pediatric disease.

[22] The rare pediatric disease designation was established as part of the pediatric voucher program in 2012. Therefore all of these designations have been granted since the program began. Of the remaining 23 requests for rare pediatric disease designations, 3 have been denied, 5 are pending review, and 15 are pending responses from the sponsors to provide additional information to enable FDA to make a final determination. In addition, there have been 5 other instances in which FDA requested information for a rare pediatric disease determination for a drug with a new drug application under review but without a designation request from a sponsor. Three of these were determined to meet the definition of a rare pediatric disease, while 1 has been denied and 1 is pending review.

[23] The financial terms for one of the voucher sales were unavailable at the time of our review.

[24] Market exclusivity generally delays marketing of generic forms of an approved product, thereby protecting its sponsor from competition for a limited period. See for example, 21 C.F.R. § 314.108 (2015).

[25] See 21 U.S.C. § 355a(b).

[26] FDA must respond within 60 days when a request for a rare pediatric disease designation is made at the same time as a request for designation of orphan disease status or fast-track designation is made. See 21 U.S.C. § 360ff(d)(2). An orphan disease designation provides incentives, such as tax credits, to the sponsor of a qualifying drug used in the diagnosis or treatment of certain rare diseases or disorders. The fast-track designation process is designed to facilitate the development and expedite the review of new drug applications to treat a broad range of serious conditions and fill an unmet medical need.

[27] While the pediatric voucher program allows drug sponsors to buy and sell vouchers that have been awarded, the government does not incur costs associated with the sale of the vouchers. Costs associated with administering the program are intended to be covered by a user fee that drug sponsors pay FDA upon redemption of a voucher.

[28] 21 U.S.C. 360ff(b)(5). This provision was subsequently amended to provide that such authority terminates effective October 1, 2016. Pub. L. No. 114-113, § 765, 129 Stat. 2242, 2287.

[29] See FDA, Rare Pediatric Disease Priority Review Vouchers, Guidance for Industry, Draft Guidance.

End Note for Appendix II

[1] The National Institutes of Health's Genetics Home Reference is available at http://ghr.nlm.nih.gov/.

INDEX

C

legislation, 10, 11, 33, 92, 118
leishmaniasis, 92
life expectancy, 32, 98, 105, 114, 116, 117
liver cells, 115, 116
liver disease, 115, 118
loss of appetite, 114

M

magnitude, 25, 46
majority, 9, 35, 40, 52, 109, 111
malabsorption, 115
malnutrition, 118
management, 5, 29, 48, 70, 96, 99, 108
manufacturing, 41, 46, 70, 80, 82
market access, 59
marketing, 5, 7, 10, 11, 12, 13, 14, 27, 33, 34, 41, 43, 54, 69, 76, 98, 119, 120
marrow, 118
Maryland, 16
measurement, 18, 24, 93
measurements, 21, 22, 66
Medicaid, 2, 40
medical, vii, 4, 6, 7, 9, 10, 11, 12, 13, 14, 15, 16, 17, 23, 37, 38, 39, 40, 41, 42, 44, 45, 49, 51, 52, 54, 55, 56, 58, 59, 62, 69, 70, 71, 72, 73, 74, 75, 78, 79, 80, 81, 82, 91, 92, 93, 96, 99, 104, 108, 112, 120
medical care, 49
Medical Device Innovation Consortium (MDIC), 2, 40, 62, 78
Medicare, 2, 40
medicine, 52
membership, 64
mental state, 66
metabolic disorder, 62, 104, 105, 115
metabolic pathways, 69
metabolism, 74
microorganisms, 119
mineralization, 117
models, 22, 23, 26, 30, 41, 50, 55, 59, 68, 69, 72, 93

molecules, 114
momentum, 41
morbidity, 13
mortality, 13, 117
multiple sclerosis, 63
muscular dystrophy, 67, 75
mutations, 14, 114

N

National Center for Advancing Translational Sciences (NCATS), 2, 47, 60, 84, 85, 89
National Center for Toxicological Research (NCTR), 2, 68, 69
National Institutes of Health, 2, 9, 84, 95, 98, 112, 113, 118, 120
National Institutes of Health (NIH), 2, 9, 28, 38, 40, 47, 48, 51, 58, 60, 61, 72, 84, 85, 87, 88, 89, 95, 98, 99, 104, 105, 112, 113, 118, 120
National Organization for Rare Disorders (NORD), 2, 15, 40, 51, 60, 78, 84, 89, 92, 112
neonates, 61, 62, 67, 80, 91
neuroblastoma, 104, 106, 114, 115
neurological disease, 60, 115
neurotoxicity, 68
New Drug Application (NDA), 2, 11
New Molecular Entity (NME), 2
Nonclinical Assessment Models (NAM), 2, 72
nutrients, 118

O

Oak Ridge Institute for Science and Education (ORISE), 3, 67, 80
obesity, 108
obstruction, 116
Office of Cellular, Tissue and Gene Therapies (OCTGT), 2, 34, 61, 85, 87
Office of Communications (OCOMM), 2, 53

P